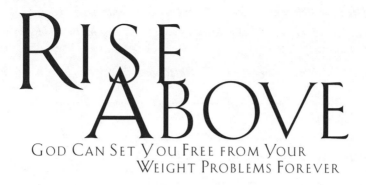

RISE ABOVE

GOD CAN SET YOU FREE FROM YOUR WEIGHT PROBLEMS FOREVER

GWEN SHAMBLIN

THOMAS NELSON PUBLISHERS®

Nashville

This book is dedicated to God and His incredible genius and to Jesus Christ and His incredible submissive walk, submissive even though He was the Son of God. Jesus had unbelievable faith to grow up knowing that He was walking straight to a cross.

Dear God, You do not get enough dedications. I pray this book brings more.

The Weigh Down Workshop, Inc.®, (and design) is a registered trademark of The Weigh Down Workshop, Inc. The Weigh Down Workshop™, Weigh Down™ (and design), and WDW™ (and design) are trademarks of The Weigh Down Workshop, Inc.

Unless otherwise noted, Scripture quotations are from the HOLY BIBLE: NEW INTERNATIONAL VERSION®. Copyright © 1973, 1978, 1984 by International Bible Society. Used by permission of Zondervan Publishing House. All rights reserved. Scripture quotations noted KJV are from the KING JAMES VERSION of the Bible.

Publisher's Note: This book is intended for general health care information only and is not intended to supplant medical advice, diagnosis, or treatment by a personal physician. Readers are urged to consult their personal physicians regarding illness, injury, and nutrition or before beginning any personal exercise program.

The photograph of the *Today's Christian Woman* cover on page 48 is by Bill Bilsley, Elgin, Illinois.

The lyrics to "Save Your Heart for Me" on page 170 are used by permission. Words and music by Gary Geld and Peter Udell. © copyright 1963 Universal-PolyGram International Publishing, Inc., a division of Universal Studios, Inc. (ASCAP). Inter-national copyright secured. All rights reserved.

ISBN 0-7852-6876-6

Printed in the United States of America.

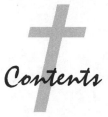

Contents

Special Thanks

You do not write a book like this without some sacrifices in the family. I have the best and most supportive family; each of you is obviously dedicated to the truth of God, and I admire you so. Thank you, David, and thank you, Michael and Michelle. You are God's Warriors.

I would like to give my thanks to The Weigh Down Workshop staff and especially to Michelle, Carole, Rob B., Joe, and Jon. I also want to thank Rob S., Teresa, Carla, Marsha, David, Rick, Jeannie, Lee, Lori, and the rest of the development staff. What incredible gifts and love you all have! The entire Weigh Down staff has been such a support—I don't know what I would have done without you and your prayers.

Finally, I would like to dedicate this book to all the frontline Weigh Down Workshop Coordinators who have fought the good fight and have advanced the kingdom of God and sought after His righteousness. I know that everything else is being added to you. March on, O Christian soldiers, as we all rise above the pull of this world!

My love and thanks to each of you,

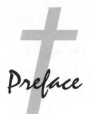

Preface

Dear Seeker,

As the Apostle Paul said,

"Everything is permissible for me"—but not everything is beneficial. "Everything is permissible for me"—but I will not be mastered by anything. "Food for the stomach and the stomach for food." (1 Cor. 6:12–13a)

You may eat anything, but you are *not* to be mastered by anything, for "you are not your own; you were bought at a price. Therefore honor God with your body" (1 Cor. 6:19b–20). To me, this sums it up. These words are straight out of the Bible, yet so many of us have a hard time implementing this simple but all-important passage. We have been mastered by food. We believe that our bodies are our own and we can do anything we want and eat any time we want. Wrong, wrong, wrong. I hope the words in this book will help you to turn this thinking around once and for all. Every line of reasoning that I have gleaned from my love of God, from the Word of God, and from the life and words of Jesus is in this book as motivation to help your heart melt before the Most High God of the universe as the Judgment Day draws near. My prayers are with you, and I want you to be encouraged as you turn toward God and away from this world.

You adulterous people, don't you know that friendship with the world is hatred toward God? Anyone who chooses to be a friend of the world becomes an enemy of God. (James 4:4)

Sincerely,

Special Considerations

If you are familiar with The Weigh Down Workshop[t] seminars and/or the book *The Weigh Down Diet,* you are aware that we recommend that you receive a medical checkup prior to beginning the program. Consulting your physician is especially vital if you have any medical condition that is impacted by foods.

Moving into the realm of "regular foods" from the grocery store, including things with salt, fat, or sugar, may be new to many of you. However, your volume of foods is going to be drastically reduced, and your body loves this! God made us sensitive to what and how much our bodies need, and you have to resurrect this system!

If you have preexisting health conditions, such as food allergies, diverticulitis, cirrhosis of the liver, diabetes, hyperlipoproteinemia, bowel resections, chronic ulcers, kidney disease, chronic constipation, and so on, make sure that you are under your physician's care and following guidelines for foods and medication. For example, if you have chronic constipation, you must keep eating fiber. If you have ulcers, take your medicine, and do not eat the foods that upset your stomach.

However, there are a few preexisting physical conditions that may be alleviated when you lose weight and start eating regular foods in smaller amounts. For example, if you have high cholesterol or triglycerides, losing weight permanently could possibly alleviate this problem. Spastic colon and ulcers could slowly improve as you eat the volume of food that your body calls for. PMS symptoms are often less intense as you lose weight. Joint and muscle problems are improved in some cases. People who are on cortisone and/or have lupus will still lose weight with no problem—it just might be a slower weight loss. You must stay in touch with your physician.

When I take medication that should be taken with food, I take it with one to three crackers. Consult your physician for what is best for you.

You are not going to believe how much energy and life you will enjoy and how much emotional improvement you will experience!

Type I and Type II Diabetes and Hypoglycemia

Consult your physician and make sure he or she is fully aware of the principles of this program if you have diabetes or hypoglycemia.

Type I diabetics need to know how to check their glucose levels regularly and to adjust insulin intake accordingly as the volume of food decreases. They must eat when their blood sugar is too low and when they feel hunger.

Type II diabetes (adult-onset) is usually the direct result of overeating. The body is overburdened by the ingestion of too much food, and the pancreas is unable to produce enough insulin to handle the excess. Diabetics who have come through the program have sometimes been able to regulate their insulin level and eliminate medication by simply reducing their intake of food, which gets the insulin/food ratio closer.

Occasionally, low blood sugar and hunger do not coincide. If blood sugar levels drop, do not panic! Usually, small amounts of food taken within a few minutes will make you feel better. This is not an open invitation to binge, however.

Introduction

If you are still struggling with losing weight, then you are not understanding this walk of death-to-self and how to accomplish it. A part of coming to God is that you humbly submit the way you have been running your life and the way you have controlled your life, and you willingly call out to Him to be the Lord of your mind and heart and soul. You invite His personality or holy attitude to come into your heart. However, you cannot do this if your own "almighty"—the god of self—is still the boss. God is not interested in a partnership because He already knows your heart, and He knows of your selfish ambition. But if you are broken enough, you will come to Him and willingly submit your old characteristics, ideas, and ways to do things, and you will let His ideas and personality rule your life. You must turn, and you must die to your will (read Rom. 5), and you must let this King rule *daily*. God has such a great personality—a personality that is *holy*. In 1 Peter 1:16, He calls us to "be holy, because I am holy." He is asking us to submit our wishes and experience His love, joy, peace, patience, kindness, and self-control leading our lives.

To stay in step with the Spirit is to *bow down* before Him. Americans have done very little of this. I praise God that I had a mother who taught me to submit to a higher authority at a young age. If you are spoiled, you will hate this more—but you *can* do it. There is no other peace on earth. This book is talking you into a death walk, a submissive walk, and a cross walk. Keep employing the Word of God in every corner of your heart, and you will begin to love this death walk because life comes from death. I am more alive than *ever before*—happier and more peaceful, blessed, patient, and loving. How? By submitting my personality to *this* personality, and I like it *much better.*

Your homework is to concentrate on this concept and put it into practice. If you do, you will find yourself permanently thin. People who do not think that we have the ability to lay down sin or to be holy have perhaps asked God into their hearts, but they have not let Him *rule.* What a King! What a Ruler! What a Boss! Let His holy personality rule in your heart, and you will experience the fruit of the Holy Spirit.

"His divine power has given us *everything* we need for life and godliness . . . so that through them *you may participate in the divine nature and escape the corruption in the world caused by evil desires"* (2 Peter 1:3–4, emphasis added).

I pray that all of you can participate in this divine personality and escape lusting after food forever.

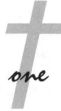

one

A PASSIONATE PEOPLE

Thank you for opening this book. I feel that God has prompted you to search deeper for the solution to the life-draining problem of extra pounds. If you are overweight, you are undoubtedly seeking deliverance from the insulting enslavement of dieting, fat gram counting, taking pills, and constantly focusing on self. Many people feel like failures and wonder why they can't seem to get their weight, their eating, and their bingeing under control. After working for years with obesity, bulimia, anorexia, and some struggling Weigh Downers, I have witnessed unprecedented weight loss success, unbelievable healing, renewed hope, and restored relationships once the principles of Weigh Down[t] were truly applied to the heart. I know that this message is God's *truth*. It is a message that will *set you free* from your struggle with food.

Many of you have already read my first book, *The Weigh Down Diet.* (If you haven't, don't despair. You will still be able to open your heart to the message presented in *Rise Above,* and you can learn more about the principles of The Weigh Down Workshop[t] by reading Appendix A and Appendix B in the back of this book.) *The Weigh Down Diet* is the skeleton of the formula for permanent weight loss. It touches on how this formula of a transferred heart can make you thin. The book explains how you can learn to stop in the middle of a candy bar and have no desire to eat the second half. God did not put rocky road ice cream or cheese dip and chips on earth to torture us; such foods are for our enjoyment. However, He wants us to learn how to rise above the magnetic pull of the excessive food, so that we do not eat more than what our body is physically calling for. Food can be an enslavement just like alcohol, tobacco, drugs, money, or any worldly pursuit that consumes our lives. The problem is the same in each case: the person's heart and passion have been given over to something other than God.

Basic Weigh Down*t*, whether in book or seminar form, teaches how to transfer this passion for food to a passion for God. It teaches that we were created with a need to be fed, both physically and spiritually. The stomach has a need to be fed with food, which the body uses as fuel in order to function physically. But for us to function emotionally and spiritually, the *heart* needs to be fed. All too often, we turn to food to feed the desires of the heart as well. However, food will never give you the true satisfaction you are looking for—it can never love you back. But as hard as it is to believe, you *can* become fulfilled by an invisible God who becomes more and more visible as you employ the suggestions made in this book. Thousands of people, some of whose testimonies you will read in this book, have done just that.

Rise Above picks up where the basic message left off. Strugglers need more motivation and heart-changing information to help them climb out of this miry pit. We all need someone and something to live for that is bigger than ourselves. We need Jesus Christ. No worldly pursuit—food, alcohol, tobacco, antidepressants, money, the praise of man, sexual lust, or whatever—will satisfy the longing heart. It is not the fault of the food, the alcohol, the money, or the tobacco. It is the effort to use them to fulfill a need that only God

Two types of holes—two types of hunger

can satisfy that is the problem. A person who eats beyond what the body is physically calling for is bound for being overweight. A person who pursues an overindulgence of alcohol, cigarettes, shopping, or power will inevitably suffer the consequences of greed. There is nothing inherently evil about food, alcohol, tobacco, money, or credit cards. In fact, it is wrong to falsely accuse God and say that the things He has approved and given on earth for good use or our enjoyment are evil. First Timothy 4:1–6 shows you exactly what God thinks of people who don't have a clue about what is right and what is wrong:

> *The Spirit clearly says that in later times some will abandon the faith and follow deceiving spirits and things taught by demons. Such teachings come through hypocritical liars, whose consciences have been seared as with a hot iron. They forbid people to marry and order them to abstain from certain foods, which God created to be received with thanksgiving by those who believe and who know the truth. For everything God created is good, and nothing is to be rejected if it is received with thanksgiving, because it is consecrated by the word of God and prayer. If you point these things out to the brothers, you will be a good minister of Christ Jesus, brought up in the truths of the faith and of the good teaching that you have followed.*

This Scripture points out that demons and people with "deceiving spirits" teach you that certain foods are evil or wrong. So the food is *not* evil. There are no "good" foods or "bad" foods (Mark 7:19; Ps. 104:14–15). If you don't realize that your being overweight is not the food's fault, you will never get out of the deep pit of obesity because you will be concentrating on the wrong thing and blaming the wrong thing. The foods are not evil; the problem is the greedy heart of man. We want more than our share.

The solution to being overweight is to go back to a reliance upon God and a trust in Him instead of all the man-made rules that have inundated our society in the last few decades and have left us increasingly heavier. According to the American Dietetic Association, one-third of the population is obese,[1] and many more are overweight. At the rate we are going, one-half of the population will be obese in the next twenty years. It is not genetic, it is not congenital, it is not inherited, it is not a disease, and it is not our mothers' fault anymore.

Due to man-made rules, America has been encouraged to lust after food. The dieter is asked to think about food content, consider the fat gram count, examine food pictures, discuss food and recipes in support groups, depend upon the scales (a focus on body and self), and prepare special meals. This focus on food makes it irresistible, for you fall in love with what you focus on. It would be like telling an alcoholic to examine all the alcoholic drinks, memorize the ingredients, drink only low-alcohol-content beverages, look at pictures of low-alcohol-content drinks, meet with support groups that discuss low-alcohol-content beverages and sample them all, hand out recipes for making your own concoctions, and then expect the addicted person to be less addicted or to abstain or drink in moderation at ten o'clock at night when no one else is around. Impossible. You fall in love with what you lust after.

This worship of food has robbed us of emotional stability, comfortable clothing, and many relationships. The solution that was introduced in *The Weigh Down Diet* is to trust God with the way He made our bodies. He has created the instincts of all animals, all infants, all children, all men, and all women with the ability to sense when they have eaten too much. Man-made rules have unplugged and confused this instinct to sense fullness and appropriate volume, and they have caused us to be greedier and to expect more self-indulgence than ever before. Dieting, which is the use of man-made rules, works only on making the *food* behave—not the heart of man. This is *big!* All animals, infants, and children that have been untouched by the man-made rules still have the strong innate capacity to recognize and respond to correct volumes of food. Dieting—including fat gram counting, pills, bulimia, suction-assisted lipectomies, and excessive exercise—has created and exacerbated an excused greed that has grown to monumental heights in this country. Greed is at its zenith. Our plates of low-calorie, fat-free foods are larger, our demand for more has increased, the seats are larger, and the clothes are stretchier. The present volume that can be eaten in polite company would have been completely embarrassing at one point in our history. Do you know what else? The word *binge* is understood by even young children. It's a word that rolls off our tongues on a daily basis with no guilt.

We are not lacking for information now; we are hurting for *motivation* and heart-changing cultivation to employ God's plan for permanent weight control. This is the book to keep by your bedside for morning motivation, to keep on your desk at work for heart-grabbing temptations, to keep in the kitchen to convict you into a whole-hearted response to the heavenly Father, and to leave by the nighttime reading chair for tearful conviction. It is full of Scripture that will soften your heart, make you satisfied with less, and therefore bring you to permanent weight control.

A major goal of this book is to introduce a holy fear of God. I am convinced this is a foundational characteristic in my heart that has moved me to obedience. Jesus delighted in the fear of God (Isa. 11:3); it cleared His mind and His path for doing God's will daily. Second Corinthians 5:10–11a says, "For we must all appear before the judgment seat of Christ, that each one may receive what is due him for the things done while in the body, whether good or bad. Since, then, we know what it is to fear the Lord, we try to persuade men." I pray the words in this book will help you develop this holy fear. I truly live for that one day called Judgment Day, and my prayer is that instead of being a dreadful day for me, this day will be romantically delightful, like a bride meeting a groom (Rev. 21:2). I picture it as a huge reception hall with everyone dressed in the most elaborate clothing. The King will spot me as I enter and allow me to walk into His presence, seeing Him face-to-face.

You are not a failure. You are a prize to be won, and there are two contenders for your heart: food (the world) and the invisible jealous God. We are a passionate people—that is why we will see people anywhere from twenty to three hundred pounds or more overweight. This represents our longing, our passion, and our lust. We salivate for more. Passion is not the problem. Our problem is *where* we direct our passion and our hearts, and where we are grabbing for more.

Dear weary ones, God can make you thin. Don't give up. Our problem is that we have swallowed the lie that says because we have been created and we now breathe, we deserve more. We can ask for more, my friends, but we must wait on our good God to provide it. Grabbing for more will depress us, will frustrate us, will kill us. James 1:14–15 tells us, "But each one is tempted when, by his own evil desire, he is dragged away and enticed. Then, after desire has conceived, it gives birth to sin; and sin, when it is full-grown, gives birth to death." But *waiting* on God to decide when and how much to feed us will bring life—the opposite of death—plus a thin body due to less greed in the heart. God knows you will feel better thin because He designed your body that way.

It's not about us—it's about God. I now get up every day and ask God, "What do *You* want me to do today?" When I consider myself and my wishes and my wants as secondary and put God's first, He takes care of me. Nothing is sweeter than knowing that someone is considering your wishes and your wants, and it is far sweeter than grabbing for and taking care of your own self. I can testify again and again to this truth. This basic law will radically transform your entire life, and your eating is the place to start testing, employing, and plastering this concept into your heart and mind.

Whether or not you are familiar with the foundational principles of the Weigh Down Workshop† program please take the time now to refresh your memory by referring to Appendix A and Appendix B before reading chapters 1 and 2, which will give you a firsthand look at how God led me to develop the Weigh Down† seminar, and how He has guided us through a true media explosion!

two

AMERICA HAS A CRUSH ON FOOD

You may have been in Weigh Down† for years or you may have just started by choosing to read this book, but I believe it would help you to know the story behind Weigh Down†. It is a story put together by the genius heavenly Father, and I couldn't see all the pieces or purposes for Weigh Down† until I looked backward. God has done some amazing things to show His power (2 Tim. 3:5).

SEEING GOD IN EVERYTHING

The way God was able to coordinate everything in nature was awesome to me! I could observe His incredible genius simply by looking at His creative ideas in our two-acre backyard in Memphis, Tennessee. I was just wowed by how God decorated the backs of ladybugs and the way He made color and fragrance come out of the ground in the form of a flower. How in the world did He put lights on the backs of bugs in the evening sky?

When I was studying for my undergraduate degree in dietetics and my master's degree in nutrition, I realized that due to my faith in a personal and caring God, I fundamentally disagreed with some of the conclusions I was taught. My belief was that God had designed every aspect of life in each and every animal. Even the personalities and senses of humor were programmed by God. Cats were snobby, and dogs were happy-go-lucky and without a chip on their shoulders.

My faith was strong enough to believe that He was the genius behind digestion and absorption. After all, God knows exactly what happens to a peanut butter and jelly sandwich after you swallow it. I questioned some of the major theories that were being taught at the time. "You are what you eat" happens to be the direct opposite of God's Word: "So do not worry, saying, 'What shall we eat?' or 'What shall we drink?' or 'What shall we wear?'" (Matt. 6:31). The food that God programmed to be desired by each animal is such genius. It allows for enough food for all the animals, and it keeps the environment clean.

Look at the animals in the wild; they are born knowing and desiring the food that they need for perfect health. The cows know to eat grass, and they know exactly how much food to eat. The birds of the air know what food they should eat, and God assigns them different menus. For example, the robin is drawn to worms, while the mockingbird likes grasshoppers. The woodpecker is programmed by God to eat bugs out of the tree. None of these birds go to bed at night and get horizontal, saying, "I really overdid it on the worms today." No. They have no greed or fear that God will not feed them the next day, so they do not overeat. Ants are taught by God to store up food for the winter, but have you ever seen an obese ant? The answer is, of course, no!

So, the "you are what you eat" theory, or the idea that we are to worry about what we should eat or drink, seemed exaggerated to me. After all, Matthew 6:25a states, "Therefore I tell you, do not worry about your life, what you will eat or drink."

Another theory I questioned was that we are genetically overweight and that dieting is the answer to obesity. I was an overeater when I was in college, and I battled weight constantly. I ate so many raw vegetables that it was the beginning of a spastic colon for me. My blouse bulged, and my pants were held together by two safety

Mary Sexton
Springfield, IL
Lost 186 lbs.
from a
beginning
weight of
almost
600 lbs.
and still
losing!

Carole Hopkins
Dyersburg, TN
Lost 150 lbs.
Has kept
it off
4 years

Virginia Schnacky
Bloomington, MN
Lost 141 lbs.
Has kept
it off
4 years

Rita Domitro
Franklin Park, IL
Lost 137 lbs.

Michele Davis
Lake Elsinore, CA
Lost 120 lbs.

Diane Bayer
Liberty, MO
Lost 125 lbs.

pins linked together because I couldn't button them. I was miserable. The rotation of diets was making me sick and frustrated, and yet the scales kept climbing.

Dietetics is basically the study of food and its impact on the body. Physicians and dietitians have been gifted with much wisdom in the areas of foods and diseases. But this wisdom was lacking in the area of permanent weight loss, as shown by statistics that indicated Americans were just getting fatter and fatter. Hospital staffing was so limited that dietitians and physicians left weight loss up to the lay public. There was an outpouring of remedies and concoctions provided by the get-rich-quick, fly-by-night entrepreneurs, many of whom had never entered a chemistry class, much less a biochemistry class. The general agreement among dietitians was that dieting and exercise were the answer. But not for me. Making the food behave by pulling out the fat or the calories was not making an impact on my overeating at all. In fact, it was only aggravating the problem.

A REVOLUTIONARY APPROACH

By the late 1970s, I attempted something revolutionary for an American: I threw away dieting, exchange lists, and low-calorie foods. I was scared of pills anyway, and I was discouraged by the exertion reward ratio of aerobics. I replaced these efforts (which was almost like giving up religion) with imitating the behavior of thin eaters, people who are not in love with food and therefore approach food differently. It seemed natural to me to study a subject from the way God made it.

My eyes were opened, and I began to see this behavior in many people. The first major behavior that I could imitate was cutting a regular meal in half. I thought that imitating the behavior of the thin eater was the major missing element. I lost all my weight, married, and went through three pregnancies, always returning to the same size that I am now. In fact, I am smaller now than I was in high school. It began to dawn on me that I had been eating only between the parameters of *hunger* and *fullness*. (More information on hunger and fullness can be found in Appendix A.)

I was certain that people were just missing this hunger and fullness information. (You have to remember that this was back in the late 1970s and early 1980s.) So I started a small group weight loss class. But just like dieting, giving people *new rules* did not make their hearts desire less food. Most of the people lost weight temporarily, but then started gaining their weight back. This was no different from the dieting statistics. Yet all I knew at this point was that I was having more and more difficulty identifying with the overeater because the thought of overeating was becoming repulsive to me. The desire to binge was disappearing, but at this point in time, I could not talk other people out of this passionate binge cycle.

THE SPIRITUAL ELEMENT

By 1986, I was at a loss and down on my knees, begging God to show me why I had no cravings for large servings, in-between-meal snacks, and late-night binges. I was gravitating toward kid-size meals, lunch servings, and getting full from just half a sandwich. Believe me, it was freaking me out, too! I was beginning to wonder if it was genetic and if I had just experienced a gene transfer. Trying to help others was my driving force, and I knew I had discovered a major key— hunger and fullness—but there had to be something else to help others achieve what I achieved with practically no pain.

Just as cutting the food in half was not the key, neither was bringing people to the realization of hunger and fullness going to be the key. But then the answers to my prayers started coming in. It took me years of constant prayers and attentiveness toward God to learn what I know today. The key to permanent weight control lies not in cutting the food in half, not in hunger and fullness; the key to permanent weight loss lies in the heart of man. Yes, something needs to change, but it is not the salad dressing or the source of meat. It is not increasing herbs, vitamins, or other concoctions. It is not messing with your metabolism or increasing your energy output, and it is not signing up for one more suction-assisted lipectomy. It is simply *eating less food* or not being *greedy* for food. I am well aware that the concept is simple, but the heart of man is complicated, and it is only unlocked and saved by its Creator: God Almighty. And that is why I have written this second book to try to expose and redirect this complex heart of man.

To start with, you need to know that we are all born to love. When I have been interviewed on secular TV programs such as *20/20* and *Larry King Live* and by newspapers such as the *Washington Post,* the interviewers would always ask, "Is this program only for the religious?" I would always answer, "We are all religious because religion is simply defined as what we give our hearts to." Religion is simply what we adore. We have all given our hearts to something because we cannot help doing that. Some have given their hearts to adore football: they know all the statistics, they know all the players, they never miss a game, and they live for the competitions. Their hearts are into it, so it is easy to want to know more and more about the sport. Others have chosen to bow down to money and will run over anyone or anything to get it. They love it; they can never get enough. It will save them, they think. Some have selected alcohol as the object of their affection; they can even get to the point that they will rob their children's piggy banks to get more of it. Some have put their hope and trust in gambling, while others have embraced sexual lust. The allure fills their day; they can't imagine a day without it. Their lives would be a bore, they think. We have the choice to give our hearts, strength, and minds to anything, and that is the basis of religion. Religion is simply what we adore, and this adoration, if it is misplaced, can have grave consequences.

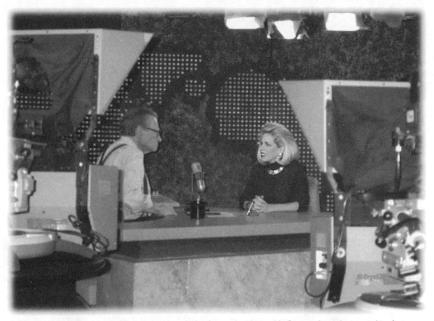

Millions watched as Larry King spent an entire hour chatting with Gwen about her passion for God, informing the nation that religion is simply what we adore. Phone lines into the Weigh Down call center were overloaded!

THE ROOT PROBLEM OF BEING OVERWEIGHT

Likewise, many Americans have given their hearts to food. Indeed, the root problem is that we are in love with food. Until we admit that we are in love—heart, soul, mind, and strength—with food, we can never lose the weight permanently. Before I lose you and you think, *Wait a minute, that's not my problem. I'm just eating the wrong food,* or *I just need to exercise more,* stay with me a little longer. Let's think about what love is.

Think back to a time when you had a crush on a guy in high school. What did you do? Well, you dressed for him, and you would plan secret rendezvous with him. You hear the voice of the one you love, so you would hear his voice over and above the hallway chatter. You would think about him in the middle of the night. Thoughts of being with him would get you out of bed in the morning. You would think about him all the time. That is a crush, and that is the behavior of a person in love.

America has a crush on food. Many of God's children have a crush on food. Why, you dress for it. You put on your stretch clothes to make sure that nothing hinders you from that rendezvous with the refrigerator at ten o'clock at night. It is a love affair with food. And just as you don't want your children or anyone else present on your rendezvous with your lover, your children had better not get up from bed and interrupt your ten o'clock binge or rendezvous with food. You hear the voice of the one you love. Even at work, you hear the popcorn popping three departments away, over and above the hubbub of the office.

All of your senses are alive to food. You can smell it, and when you go to parties, you don't really care about the company—just the buffet. Food is what you think about to help you get out of bed. You can get through the morning at work if you can just get to lunch. You can put in a good afternoon's work as long as you reward yourself

Dinner becomes an all-evening love affair.

with your anticipated five to ten o'clock din-ner—you know, the one that begins with hitting the refrigerator as soon as you get home, eating dinner as you cook it, sitting down to eat with the family, and picking at the leftovers. And then there is the snack as you watch late-night TV. *You see, when you've lusted after food all day long, your heart has* no choice *but to spend the evening with your lover.*

OUR AMERICAN INHERITANCE

The truth we are trying to establish is that you were born to love, and you have an opportunity on earth to choose what you love. It is no wonder so many of us have selected food as the object of our affec-tion. We come by it naturally—in fact, it's been handed down. Many of our great-grandparents, grandparents, and parents have passed down this reverence for food. For example, early in life, mothers with their babies have force-fed the bottle, even if the baby is rejecting the last few ounces of milk. We have felt obligated to serve the bottle, not the baby. It seems so innocent, but to do this action, we have to have more faith in the food than we do in God. There's hope that the milk will give that baby health, so the mother is desperate to get it down the baby. There are hope in and dependence on the food, instead of confidence in God's incredibly well-designed natural system.

The truth we are trying to establish is that you were born to love, and you have an opportunity on earth to choose what you love.

By the time our babies are toddlers, we resort to making airplane games out of the food to coax them into finishing it. Once again, we cater more to what the food industry considers a serving size than to the child's God-given internal control. That is a lack of faith.

The result has been that we have successfully unplugged the hunger mechanism for the next generation. As a child, you knew that you had better run to the table while the food was hot because it was more important than you or what you were doing. Once you were at the table, there were all those food rules: "Don't play with your food." "You had better not waste your food." "You can't have dessert until you've finished everything on your plate." More always seemed to be better, and most mothers were members of the "clean your plate" club. Some of these table rules could be very innocent. But you know there are families who make it obvious that by the end of the eating experience, the food has been elevated to a position high enough that you have to jump through hoops for it. At the end of the meal, you make sure that the leftovers are stored in the finest of Tupperware containers and refrigerated at forty-five degrees because you don't want the food to go bad.

Yes, it is handed down; so in a sense, it is inherited, but it is *not* genetic. The answer to obesity will be found not in the genes, as scientists are trying to establish, but in the heart—or spirit—of man. It is a chosen spiritual addiction, and we pass the legacy of our idols down to our children. Your children can see that the thought of food lights up your eyes. Scripture backs this up. In Exodus 20:1–6, you see the generational forecast:

And God spoke all these words: "I am the LORD your God, who brought you out of Egypt, out of the land of slavery. You shall have no other gods before me. You shall not make for yourself an idol in the form of anything in heaven above or on the earth beneath or in the waters below. You shall not bow down to them or worship them; for I, the LORD your God, am a jealous God, punishing the children for the sin of the fathers to the third and fourth generation of those who hate me, but showing love to a thousand generations of those who love me and keep my commandments."

As a consequence of adopting the family's focus, food (in its storage form) accumulated on our hips and on our gut. The family's reverence had us bowing down to the refrigerator, and now we were beginning to look like one. In other words, we accumulated the meat

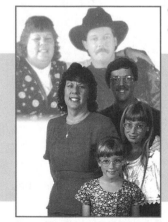

drawer on one hip and the freezer on the other hip. We put the dairy section in our

I have been overweight for 17 years, and at one point, I gained 100 pounds in one year, reaching 300 pounds. My husband, John, has also been overweight most of his life, and our children's lives were being affected by our lifestyles. We have tried man's ways to lose weight, but now John, our two girls, and I have accepted Jesus Christ as our Lord and Savior, and He has completely changed our lives!
Karen Clayburn—Denver, CO

Karen Clayburn lost 178 pounds. John Clayburn lost 56 pounds. They accepted Christ through teachings of truth found in Weigh Down.†

stomachs, and then we packed in the leftovers behind us! We never dreamed that we would wind up like this.

DIETING: THE COUNTERFEIT SALVATION FOR OBESITY

In desperation, we turned to man and man-made rules for the answer. We needed a Savior—desperately. We were in it deep. By the early 1960s and especially by the 1970s, local weight loss groups popped up on every corner, and diets were as numerous as the sands on the seashore. We were looking for a liberator from this disgusting overweight condition. A portion of the population moved to throwing up and anorexia, while the rest of the population poured out their life savings on the diet of the month. But man-made rules will never work. The Bible dispels man-made rules as a means of saving us, and our coordinated God wants to be our Savior.

A foundational Scripture of Weigh Down† is Colossians 2:16a, 20–23. There is a great deal to be learned from this passage as you study it closely:

> *Therefore do not let anyone judge you by what you eat or drink. . . . Since you died with Christ to the basic principles of this world, why, as though you still belonged to it, do you submit to its rules: "Do not handle! Do not taste! Do not touch!"? These are all destined to perish with use, because they are based on human commands and teachings. Such regulations indeed have an appearance of wisdom, with their self-imposed worship, their false humility and their harsh treatment of the body, but they lack any value in restraining sensual indulgence.*

Not only do man-made rules not help with indulgence; they compound the problem, proving to be an incubator for cultivating a deeper love relationship with food than we would have had if we had never, ever dieted.

Why has dieting been such an incubator? We fall in love with what we focus on. It's a simple fact. That's how your kids fall in love with rock stars or sports figures. They know all the players and all the statistics, and they put posters on the wall. We're no different. Look at this incubator. The more we dieted, the more we focused on what we should eat and what we should not eat. Dieting forced us to spend hours reading labels, planning meals, looking at and lusting after foods, and counting the calories we were burning in order to calculate the calories we could eat. We got up every morning thinking, *What am I going to eat, and what am I not going to eat?* After preparing our own lists, we went to work and asked others what they were going to eat and what they were not going to eat. We had to focus on where we were going for lunch because not just any restaurant would let us boil our packages of dehydrated food. During the Sunday morning sermon, we dreamed of where we were going for the Sunday lunch buffet. We scrutinized menus for low-fat meals. And when the next diet book came out, we bought it. We were no longer cooking one meal in the evening—we had to cook two: one for the family and one for ourselves.

The result? This passed-down reverence for food plus this dieting incubator, which made us even more focused and therefore infatuated with food, equal a widespread epidemic of obesity. The *Journal of the American Medical Association* stated that more than 50 percent of American adults are overweight.[1] According to the American Dietetic Association, 33 percent of Americans are *obese,* which means they are 20 percent over their ideal body weight.[2] One recent article in *Healthy Kids* magazine stated that 30 to 40 percent of America's children are overweight or obese.[3] Europe and Canada are quickly catching up with the United States. People are putting on weight faster than ever before. According to the most conservative estimates, at the rate we are going, half of the American population will be overweight in the next twenty years. It is America's number one health problem and the single most-related factor to early death.[4]

According to these statistics, if you are not fat now, the odds are that you will be. If you still don't believe this is an epidemic, think about it— even though animals have the strong innate ability to sense what they should eat, we have nonetheless placed our pet dogs and our cats on low-fat diets!

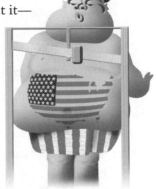

We have built an entire culture based on studying the content of food. We have examined its moral character under a microscope, and yet we have not studied the motives of our own hearts at all. We are experts at reading labels. We even know how many calories are used when

Passed-down reverence for food + dieting incubator = America's epidemic of obesity

we talk on the phone. However, what we didn't know was that this growing preoccupation of fat grams and labels would enslave our hearts in direct proportion to our infatuation with the food and diets. It is a spiritual cancer much like a slow-growing physical cancer that overtakes human organs, or an insidious addiction that has slowly engulfed your very life.

You see, obesity is the result of having a spiritual enslavement to food, impacting far more than just the size of our clothes. Many people I have counseled have seriously considered suicide, and family life is adversely affected by this focus. We wanted a way out of this enslavement, and at first, dieting looked like the solution. All dieters think they are just one diet away from turning it around. After a while, however, gaining and losing become secondary to the euphoria that comes from bingeing on the food. But this is inevitably followed by depression when the binge ends. To counteract this depression, the overeater starts yet another diet, which leads to a greater focus on the slave master called food. This only makes the heart sink deeper into the clutches of food and overweight.

As you can see, in spite of its hard labor and empty pocketbooks,

America is enslaved. It is enslaved at the rate of an extra two and a half pounds per person per year. America has placed its hope in the diet, its faith in the diet, and its heart in the food.

Many years ago, when I saw in Scriptures that it is not the food's fault (Mark 7:14–19; Col. 2:16–23; 1 Tim. 4:1–5; Heb. 13:9) and that the problem was the heart of man (Phil. 3:17–19; Mark 7:19; Ex. 20), God was also showing me the symbolism of the Exodus story (see Appendix B). Enslavement to a master other than God—whether it is food calling your name and commanding your attention or sex controlling you and occupying your heart and mind—is still enslavement. Enslavement is a part of our nature. We are all attached or enslaved to something, and we are good slaves. But food will never love you back. You are embracing something that is draining the life out of you. Think about it. We read in the book of Exodus that God's children, the Israelites, were in bondage to a wicked master, the pharaoh of Egypt, who did not care whether they lived or died.

If you are enslaved to food, then I promise that food will damage your body. Overeating is the number one cause of death. How many eighty- or ninety-year-olds do you see who are overweight? Gorging yourself is killing your kidneys, liver, heart, and joints. It is straining your emotions, robbing you of happiness, and depressing you every day. Bowing down to ice cream, crackers, fast food, and potato chips is enslaving. I know you want out. Studying the following chapter will help you to see how the God of the universe delivers and moves and thinks. You do not want to miss *your* exodus from obesity and dieting.

What You Can Do Today

➤ *Go where God is leading you in Scripture.*

➤ *Comprehend the seriousness of your enslavement to food.* Understand that depending upon food for comfort, enjoyment, entertainment, friendship, romance, or anything but sustenance is depending upon an idol or a false god. The Bible refers to this as *idolatry,* and the two major concepts condemned throughout the Bible are idolatry and adultery. Both show contempt and greed because the offender is rejecting the object for which it was made to love or to marry. The Bible says that greed is idolatry (Col. 3:5), and this is understandable because the greedy person has left God and is depending upon another god. God is far too jealous to allow this type of lusting relationship with food to continue. He deserves for us—and expects us—to keep our covenant relationship with Him pure and undefiled. Please contemplate the following passages until you comprehend the seriousness of this misplaced dependence and passion: Ezekiel 22:3–5; 23:48; and Deuteronomy 32:20–22.

➤ *Think about how your family considers food.* At mealtime, is the food more important than the people sitting around the table? Does your family enforce food rules, such as cleaning your plate before you can have dessert? Talk with your family tonight, and make some changes in the way food has controlled your time together.

➤ *Find someone who is not in love with food: a thin eater.* Start observing how thin eaters approach their eating occasions. Notice that they are not controlled by the food.

➤ *Think about all the diets and man-made eating rules you have followed in the past.* Recognize how useless they were at changing your heart. Realize that God is not going to let any of these man-made plans be your savior.

Feasting on the Will of the Father

At the end of each chapter, I will describe how I approach different eating occasions. If you find yourself lusting after the foods that I am describing, just turn the page and that will stop the problem. Lusting is a major root of obesity; we must not let ourselves go there.

When I was struggling with weight, I approached food prayerfully. I am always talking to God. He loves that, and He lets me know because He answers prayers. Answered prayer is the key to finding this relationship with God, but it comes only by way of a journey.

First, realize that God is calling you to purity (1 Tim. 4:12), holiness (Heb. 12:14), and righteousness (Matt. 5:6). You must seek His kingdom and His righteousness *first* (this is deep). Matthew 6:33 says, "But seek first his kingdom and his righteousness, and all these things will be given to you as well." Notice it says *"His* righteousness"—doing what *He* thinks is right. We must stay in the Word until His wishes are second nature. After all, He is the Boss and we are employees. It isn't about performance—it is an attitude.

Second, when you abide in Jesus this way, He promises that your prayers will be answered: "If you remain in me and my words remain in you, ask whatever you wish, and it will be given you" (John 15:7). "This is the confidence we have in approaching God: that if we ask anything according to his will, he hears us" (1 John 5:14). I ask in the name of Jesus that I will be able to find my keys, get through traffic, and pick out something great to eat, wear, and serve at a party. God is *so fun!*

Discovering His great ability to comfort, care, direct, and guide is my zeal. From this overflow, I write, speak, and sing to help others find the path to getting every prayer answered. When I approach food, I'm prayerful, thankful, and full of joy toward this Genius of recipes. This fullness prevents me from desiring extra food. Keep reading because I have much more to share! *For whoever finds me finds life and receives favor from the LORD* (Prov. 8:35).

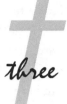

three

THE EXODUS SYMBOLISM

America is actually in the middle of Egypt, and it doesn't even know it. Like the Israelites, we have invested our energy in Egypt (see Appendix B for Egyptian symbolism). Just as the Israelites became professional brick makers, we have become professional dieters. We have let the food become our master. We have let it call our names and summon us from the pantry, and we have then become enslaved to the ensuing constant dieting, eating tasteless foods, counting calories, counting fat grams, and becoming obsessed with exercise and bulimia. The Israelites built pyramids, but we have built relationships with the kitchen and have built weight loss institutions across the world. We have acted as if God has forsaken the land. The coins that we have inscribed with "In God We Trust" have been used to pay for Egyptian (worldly) remedies and concoctions to get us out of this mess. When the white coats told us that the answer was in the form of a pill, we bought it and we swallowed it. Then when they told us the answer was in the form of a liquid, we emptied our pocketbooks and guzzled it. Then when they told us the answer was stomach stapling and suction-assisted lipectomies, we took out a loan and tried them. These remedies have not "saved" us from loving food.

The Israelites stayed in Egypt for 430 years, and then they cried out for a Savior. America has been in a mess for decades, and we have cried out to God again and again to remove this fat and save us from this burden. Does it surprise us that after we have finally lost faith in the world's methods—only after recycling the same diet one hundred times, of course—we turn to God? That is just like mankind—we resort to God instead of making Him first. After 430 years, it would seem to the Israelites that God had deserted the land—and after years of obesity and dieting, it would seem to us that God has deserted us. But of course, He hasn't! However, just as He didn't respond until the children of Israel wanted out and cried out for a Savior, He will not respond until we want to be saved from the enslavement of food! We have to ask ourselves: Do we really want out of this relationship with food?

> Does it surprise us that after we have finally lost faith in the world's methods—only after recycling the same diet one hundred times, of course—we turn to God? That is just like mankind—we resort to God instead of making Him first.

For some, it may take 430 years of repetitive bricklaying—that is, using the same diets over and over—to be convinced to call out to God. God knows that it takes a response from the bottom of our hearts to want out of the love of food. Otherwise, when He reaches down to save us, it is like pulling a twelve-month-old away from his mother. The baby would want to go right back to the mother's arms. Wanting out puts many things into motion.

In Genesis 46:4a, God spoke these words: "I will go down to Egypt with you, and I will surely bring you back again." Even though God was talking to Jacob, He is talking to us today. Why would God want us to go to Egypt? Well, I look at it this way: God is so good-looking, so athletic, so powerful, and so charming that upon first sight, we would all immediately bow down and adore Him. So He made Himself invisible to make the contest a little more fair. On top of that, He is such a humble gentleman that He took us to Egypt and allowed us to meet His rival face-to-face. Although God did not allow us to touch, see, or hear Him, He put us in the middle of His competition and allowed us to use every sense to experience it. In other words, He let us taste the world and flirt with the world, but unfortunately, some of us have become married to the world. That was the chance that God was willing to take. He didn't want us to wind up in heaven and in His arms without a choice, never having "dated around," so to speak. God wasn't going to lock us up in some castle where we couldn't see the opponent. He's a gentleman. As good-looking as He is and as athletic as He is, He is not going to let Himself be visible because He knows that we would all bow down and worship Him immediately. There is no competition—there is no one else in His league. So, yes, He is going to let us "date around"—that's Plan A—so we can appreciate what a great choice He is. But unfortunately, some of His children—in fact, a *lot* of His children—have lost their focus and become distracted, and therefore found their hearts enslaved to Egypt, with no idea of how to get out of this relationship. This was not part of Plan A. So God had to resort to Plan B: a duel—a boxing match—a fight.

God's fight would be with the pharaoh of Egypt and with the one whom Pharaoh symbolizes, Satan. Satan, or the devil, is a very powerful spiritual being whom many people do not take seriously. Some see him as a cartoon character with a pitchfork. Others imagine him as a repulsive creature they have seen in a horror movie. But the Bible teaches that Satan and his angels rebelled against his heavenly Father and were cast out of heaven (Rev. 12:7–8).

God has allowed Satan to roam the earth and compete for the hearts and minds of the people. Ephesians 6:11–12 says that the devil is the leader of the spiritual forces of evil. Sometimes Satan is very direct, as in the biblical incidents of demon possession or the time he murdered Job's family by causing a windstorm and caused the financial ruin of Job's estate (Job 1). Other times, particularly when he

God wasn't going to lock us up in some castle where we couldn't see the opponent. He's a gentleman. As good-looking as He is and as athletic as He is, He is not going to let Himself be visible because He knows that we would all bow down and worship Him immediately.

wants us to follow him, he is more covert or deceptive, as when he lied to Adam and Eve about the consequences of eating from the one and only tree that God had clearly forbidden. Satan also is the source of temptation, which people give in to through their own lack of self-control (1 Cor. 7:5), doing what is sinful or evil (1 John 3:8). And the consequences of sin are devastating—as in the poor health or death that results from overindulgence in food. But we have the power, through devotion to our heavenly Father and His Son, our Savior Jesus Christ, to defeat the dark force of Satan. James 4:7 states, "Submit yourselves, then, to God. Resist the devil, and he will flee from you."

In the Exodus story, God demonstrates His overwhelming power over Egypt and Egypt's master, Pharaoh, who represents Satan. God wasn't going to leave what was rightfully His in the arms and clutches of Egypt. The Israelites' backs were breaking under the strain of the labor, and they cried out to God. Once the children of God cried out to the Father from this pain, they were ready for the Exodus—one of the most incredible stories on earth.

If you, too, are crying out to our heavenly Father to save you from this heartless slave driver called food, then you are ready for the exodus as well. You are ready for salvation from the love of this earth. The problem has been that it has never occurred to us that our hearts needed to be saved or rescued. We didn't know that it was super-glued to the food. But since the key to unlocking obesity is in our hearts, it cannot be found in the nutrition books, and we must go to God's Word for answers.

THE EXODUS STORY

The Exodus story explains the unseen war for the heart's devotion. This information is the necessary information to unlock your heart from the clutches of food, alcohol, or sexual lust. It is a neglected story that should have been passed down from generation to generation. Please read on. . . .

The book of Exodus explains how a large group of God's children were saved from bowing down to an earthly ruler. It is symbolic of how God has saved many people in Weigh Down† from overweight, and it is symbolic of how God wants to save you today. The first clue that God was aware of the desperate cries of the enslaved Israelites and had not abandoned the land was when He called Moses and prepared him for action.

In Exodus 5, Moses and Aaron went to Pharaoh and told him to let God's people go to worship God in the desert. You see, you can't worship God in Egypt. You have to get out of Egypt to worship God. "Pharaoh said, 'Who is the LORD that I should obey him and let Israel go? I do not know the LORD and I will not let Israel go'" (Ex. 5:2). Then he told Moses and Aaron to get back to work and stop taking the people away from their labor.

It is interesting to note that when you have a heart for God but are enslaved by something on this earth, it is labor—it is work. Dieting is hard work: counting fat grams, measuring foods, using exchange lists, having to stick to regimented exercise routines, denying yourself the foods you really want, and more. It consumes your energy and your time. Well, it was about to get even harder on the Israelites.

That same day Pharaoh gave this order to the slave drivers and fore-men in charge of the people: "You are no longer to supply the people with straw for making bricks; let them go and gather their own straw. But require them to make the same number of bricks as before; don't reduce the quota. They are lazy; that is why they are crying out, 'Let

us go and sacrifice to our God.' Make the work harder for the men so
that they keep working and pay no attention to lies." (Ex. 5:6–9)

Have you noticed that when you finally make a decision to leave
Egypt so that you can truly worship God, Satan doubles the trouble?
He is not afraid when you are in the middle of Egypt, happily making your bricks for Pharaoh and bowing down to him—in other
words, when you're dieting, counting fat grams, and exercising
obsessively. But when you decide to leave behind your exchange lists
and pictures of food to go forward with a new focus on God, you can
be sure there will be a period when Satan doubles the labor by with-
holding the straw. Keep in mind that when you decide to leave Egypt
and worship God, you will hear people saying, "You're so gullible.
Are you really going to a quick-fix program where they are telling
you that you can eat what you want to eat? You're just looking for
the easy way out! Get to work! You need to count your fat grams
and start your exercise program again. You are just lazy."

Please don't listen to that lie. You'll never get out of Egypt if you
do. Satan will always make you feel that you are lazy and unpro-
ductive when you are developing a love relationship with God or
seeking the kingdom and His righteousness first. Never forget that
fact. You are not lazy when you are giving your heart, soul, mind,
and strength to build a love relationship with God and leave a love
relationship with this earth behind. You're not lazy at all.

Once the labor doubled, the Israelites cried out even more.
Therefore, God sent Moses and Aaron to Pharaoh. "Aaron threw his
staff down in front of Pharaoh and his officials, and it became a
snake. Pharaoh then summoned wise men and sorcerers, and the
Egyptian magicians also did the same things by their secret arts: Each
one threw down his staff and it became a snake. But Aaron's staff
swallowed up their staffs" (Ex. 7:10–12).

To make a fair, clear, obviously superior challenge, God made
Aaron's staff become a snake. The Egyptian specialists were able to

duplicate this supernatural act, just as our present-day worldly specialists are able to temporarily produce weight loss. Symbolically, just as Aaron's snake swallowed up the Egyptian snakes, God will ensure that the worldly weight loss techniques will not survive. He is swallowing them up as we speak. But Pharaoh's heart became hard, and he would not listen to them, just as God had predicted.

Now the challenge had been made. The chance for Egypt to back down without any physical damage had been offered. It was too late to go back. The fight between God and the ruler of this earth began. God is going to make a mighty distinction between Egyptians and His children—people who want to love the world versus people who want to love Him. Since Pharaoh would not listen, God was devising some penalties for Egypt.

The fight between God and the ruler of this earth began. God is going to make a mighty distinction between Egyptians and His children—people who want to love the world versus people who want to love Him.

Round One

The first round between the heavyweight champions was the plague of blood. In Exodus 7, we read the following:

The LORD said to Moses, "Tell Aaron, 'Take your staff and stretch out your hand over the waters of Egypt—over the streams and canals, over the ponds and all the reservoirs'—and they will turn to blood. Blood will be everywhere in Egypt, even in the wooden buckets and stone jars." Moses and Aaron did just as the LORD had commanded. He raised his staff in the presence of Pharaoh and his officials and struck the water of the Nile, and all the water was changed into blood. The fish in the Nile died, and the river smelled so bad that the Egyptians could not drink its water. Blood was everywhere in Egypt. . . . And all

the Egyptians dug along the Nile to get drinking water, because they
could not drink the water of the river. (vv. 19–21, 24)

Please imagine, if you can, the Nile being filled with blood. With
the heat of Egypt, the stench would be unbearable. You could not
wash in the water, and an overwhelming impact of this first plague
would be thirst. Even a small amount of blood spilled is frightening
to me, but rivers and basins and faucets of blood would be terrifying.
Anyone in his right mind would have given in, but since the Egyptian
magicians were able to make blood with their secret arts, Pharaoh's
heart was hardened.

Round Two

Before the land was purged from the color of red, Round Two
would begin.

Then the LORD said to Moses, "Go to Pharaoh and say to him, 'This
is what the LORD says: Let my people go, so that they may worship
me. If you refuse to let them go, I will plague your whole country with
frogs. The Nile will teem with frogs. They will come up into your
palace and your bedroom and onto your bed, into the houses of your
officials and on your people, and into your ovens and kneading
troughs. The frogs will go up on you and your people and all your offi-
cials.'" Aaron stretched out his hand over the waters of Egypt, and the
frogs came up and covered the land. But the magicians did the same
things by their secret arts; they also made frogs come up on the land
of Egypt. Pharaoh summoned Moses and Aaron and said, "Pray to
the LORD to take the frogs away from me and my people, and I will
let your people go to offer sacrifices to the LORD." Moses said to
Pharaoh, "I leave to you the honor of setting the time for me to pray
for you and your officials and your people that you and your houses
may be rid of the frogs, except for those that remain in the Nile."
"Tomorrow," Pharaoh said. Moses replied, "It will be as you say, so

that you may know there is no one like the LORD our God." (Ex.
8:1–4, 6–10)

So the Lord made the frogs die, and they were piled in heaps. But
once Pharaoh saw that there was relief, he hardened his heart and
would not listen to Moses and Aaron. Round Three would begin.

Round Three

In the next plague,

The LORD said to Moses, "Tell Aaron, 'Stretch out your staff and strike
the dust of the ground,' and throughout the land of Egypt the dust will
become gnats." They did this, and when Aaron stretched out his hand
with the staff and struck the dust of the ground, gnats came upon men
and animals. All the dust throughout the land of Egypt became gnats.
But when the magicians tried to produce gnats by their secret arts, they
could not. And the gnats were on men and animals. The magicians said
to Pharaoh, "This is the finger of God." But Pharaoh's heart was hard
and he would not listen, just as the LORD had said. (Ex. 8:16–19)

Yes, this was the finger of God. And just as the ancient plagues
from God resulted in thirst, slimy amphibians invading their personal space, and irritants buzzing around in their eyes, in their ears,
and in their mouths, God's finger has been working in your life and
is moving this very minute. Not only is God trying to make you
aware of His power and presence; He is actually causing discomfort.

If you don't think God works that way, look at how He dealt
with mankind in the beginning, starting with Adam and Eve. In
Eve, He increased labor pain, and with Adam, He increased the pain
of labor. Whenever we are where we are not supposed to be, God
will start with irritating, disturbing, nagging annoyances that un-
settle us. We may not have blood, frogs, and gnats, but we have
clothes that are too tight, exhaustion by 10:00 A.M., trouble breathing,

trouble sleeping, indigestion, and nagging comments. As difficult as this is, like Pharaoh, we wait until tomorrow, or even Monday, to call upon God, hoping that these annoyances will just go away without any repentance on our part.

Just as the ancient plagues from God resulted in thirst, slimy amphibians invading their personal space, and irritants buzzing around in their eyes, in their ears, and in their mouths, God's finger has been working in your life and is moving this very minute.

Up until now, these plagues had been just annoying. For some, the annoyances were painful enough that they packed their bags and left Egypt. But unfortunately for most, it would take more. And Satan, who is symbolized by Pharaoh, does not want us to stop bowing down to him, and an even more basic goal of his is to ensure that we do not bow down to God. Satan was and still is jealous for the devotion of God's children, but he is no match for God. A normal opponent would have let go in Round One, but God allowed Satan's heart to stay hardened, so that we could see more of God's passion and power—more of His passion for a good fight, more of His passion for our hearts, and more of His passion to show how distinctively different He is. Before it is over, He will demonstrate that Satan and the lure of the world (food, money, sex, etc.) don't even belong in the ring. God has no contender.

Round Four

Due to the hardening of Pharaoh's heart, we are now going to relive a different level of combat, which starts with Round Four.

> Then the LORD said to Moses, "Get up early in the morning and confront Pharaoh as he goes to the water and say to him, 'This is what the LORD says: Let my people go, so that they may worship me. If you

do not let my people go, I will send swarms of flies on you and your officials, on your people and into your houses. The houses of the Egyptians will be full of flies, and even the ground where they are. But on that day, I will deal differently with the land of Goshen, where my people live; no swarms of flies will be there, so that you will know that I, the LORD, *am in this land. I will make a distinction between my people and your people. This miraculous sign will occur tomorrow.'" And the* LORD *did this. Dense swarms of flies poured into Pharaoh's palace and into the houses of his officials, and throughout Egypt the land was ruined by the flies.* (Ex. 8:20–24)

Rounds Five and Six

Then the LORD *said to Moses, "Go to Pharaoh and say to him, 'This is what the* LORD, *the God of the Hebrews, says: "Let my people go, so that they may worship me." If you refuse to let them go and continue to hold them back, the hand of the* LORD *will bring a terrible plague on your livestock in the field—on your horses and donkeys and camels and on your cattle and sheep and goats. But the* LORD *will make a distinction between the livestock of Israel and that of Egypt, so that no animal belonging to the Israelites will die.'" . . . Pharaoh sent men to investigate and found that not even one of the animals of the Israelites had died. Yet his heart was unyielding and he would not let the people go. Then the* LORD *said to Moses and Aaron, "Take handfuls of soot from a furnace and have Moses toss it into the air in the presence of Pharaoh. It will become fine dust over the whole land of Egypt, and festering boils will break out on men and animals throughout the land." So they took soot from a furnace and stood before Pharaoh. Moses tossed it into the air, and festering boils broke out on men and animals. The magicians could not stand before Moses because of the boils that were on them and on all the Egyptians. But the* LORD *hardened Pharaoh's heart and he would not listen to Moses and Aaron, just as the* LORD *had said to Moses.* (Ex. 9:1–4, 7–12)

As you can see, God was introducing a new point by the fourth plague. And from this plague on, He spared His children from the devastation, making sure that all the world knew that those who wanted to go and worship Him were treasured and favored and beloved.

What was once an annoyance had become something far more agonizing. Those of us who did not leave Egypt after the annoyances have found that being overweight is now more than just uncomfortable; it is becoming physically damaging. What were once minor symptoms have now become chronic syndromes. Instead of festering boils, it is festering marriage difficulties and financial problems. Can it get worse if we continue to cling to a false god in our lives? I'm afraid so. God could have easily stopped here, but more needed to be established about His powerful leadership and disclosed about man's stubborn heart.

Rounds Seven and Eight

At Round Seven, God took a people who now had diseased livestock, ruined livelihoods, and bodies covered in boils, and He moved them into the full-blown fury of plagues.

"This is what the LORD, the God of the Hebrews, says: Let my people go, so that they may worship me, or this time I will send the full force of my plagues against you and against your officials and your people, so you may know that there is no one like me in all the earth. For by now I could have stretched out my hand and struck you and your people with a plague that would have wiped you off the earth. But I have raised you up for this very purpose, that I might show you my power and that my name might be proclaimed in all the earth. You still

set yourself against my people and will not let them go. Therefore, at
this time tomorrow I will send the worst hailstorm that has ever fallen
on Egypt, from the day it was founded till now. Give an order now to
bring your livestock and everything you have in the field to a place of
shelter, because the hail will fall on every man and animal that has not
been brought in and is still out in the field, and they will die." . . . So
the LORD *rained hail on the land of Egypt; hail fell and lightning*
flashed back and forth. It was the worst storm in all the land of Egypt
since it had become a nation. Throughout Egypt hail struck everything
in the fields—both men and animals; it beat down everything growing
in the fields and stripped every tree. The only place it did not hail was
the land of Goshen, where the Israelites were. (Ex. 9:13b–19, 23b–26)

Even after the Egyptians were almost beaten to death, Pharaoh's
heart got harder—something that seems unimaginable. The Bible
tells us:

So Moses and Aaron went to Pharaoh and said to him, "This is what
the LORD*, the God of the Hebrews, says: 'How long will you refuse to*
humble yourself before me? Let my people go, so that they may wor-
ship me. If you refuse to let them go, I will bring locusts into your
country tomorrow. They will cover the face of the ground so that it can-
not be seen. They will devour what little you have left after the hail,
including every tree that is growing in your fields.'" . . . So Moses
stretched out his staff over Egypt, and the LORD *made an east wind*
blow across the land all that day and all that night. By morning the
wind had brought the locusts; they invaded all Egypt and settled
down in every area of the country in great numbers. Never before had
there been such a plague of locusts, nor will there ever be again. They
covered all the ground until it was black. They devoured all that was
left after the hail—everything growing in the fields and the fruit on
the trees. Nothing green remained on tree or plant in all the land in
Egypt. . . . Pharaoh's officials said to him, "How long will this man

be a snare to us? Let the people go, so that they may worship the LORD their God. Do you not yet realize that Egypt is ruined?" . . . But the LORD hardened Pharaoh's heart, and he would not let the Israelites go. (Ex. 10:3–5, 13–15, 7, 20)

Egypt was a punching bag. As in any fight, you would hope that the referee would stop the fight when it got this one-sided, but this fight would continue.

Round Nine

Now watch what happened in the ninth round, as God took a new twist on His tactics:

Then the LORD said to Moses, "Stretch out your hand toward the sky so that darkness will spread over Egypt—darkness that can be felt." So Moses stretched out his hand toward the sky, and total darkness covered all Egypt for three days. No one could see anyone else or leave his place for three days. Yet all the Israelites had light in the places where they lived. Then Pharaoh summoned Moses and said, "Go, worship the LORD. Even your women and children may go with you; only leave your flocks and herds behind." But Moses said, "You must allow us to have sacrifices and burnt offerings to present to the LORD our God. Our livestock too must go with us; not a hoof is to be left behind." (Ex. 10:21–26a)

The Lord wants every part of our hearts to leave Egypt—not even a *hoof* must be left behind. Satan knows if a part of your heart is left behind, he will eventually have the whole heart again in his clutches. Pharaoh was mad at this request, and he was not willing to let them go. Pharaoh was so mad, in fact, that he threatened to kill Moses if he appeared before him again.

After devastating hailstorms and locusts, the Egyptians had total darkness for three days. No one could see anyone else or go anywhere. Likewise, as we keep our hearts in Egypt and insist on worshiping food or anything in this world, we become increasingly robbed relationally and financially, so that anything green in our lives is destroyed. Like Pharaoh, we do not yet realize that Egypt is ruined—that our lives are miserable. Eventually, it leads to spiritual blackness. A blackness that can be felt. A separation from the light and love of God is the most fearful plague. Just as they could not leave their houses, many of us today have become confined to our own houses by panic attacks and other fears. We can't seem to lift our heads to worship anything.

Satan knows if a part of your heart is left behind, he will eventually have the whole heart again in his clutches.

Finally, the last category is death. In the final round, God pulled a right hook on Egypt—the final blow, the knockout punch.

Round Ten

Now the LORD had said to Moses, "I will bring one more plague on Pharaoh and on Egypt. After that, he will let you go from here, and when he does, he will drive you out completely." ... So Moses said, "This is what the LORD says: 'About midnight I will go throughout Egypt. Every firstborn son in Egypt will die, from the firstborn son of Pharaoh, who sits on the throne, to the firstborn son of the slave girl, who is at her hand mill, and all the firstborn of the cattle as well. There will be loud wailing throughout Egypt—worse than there has ever been or ever will be again. But among the Israelites not a dog will bark at any man or animal.' Then you will know that the LORD makes a distinction between Egypt and Israel." ... At midnight the LORD struck down all the firstborn in Egypt, from the firstborn of Pharaoh, who sat on the throne, to the firstborn of the prisoner, who was in the dungeon, and the firstborn of all the livestock as well. (Ex. 11:1, 4–7; 12:29)

The Israelites were instructed not to go out of their doors until morning. And as the Lord went through the land to strike down the Egyptians, He saw the blood on the tops and sides of the door-frames. He passed over those doorways and did not permit the destroyer to enter those houses. "Pharaoh and all his officials and all the Egyptians got up during the night, and there was loud wailing in Egypt, for there was not a house without someone dead" (Ex. 12:30).

The children of God were spared because they had sprinkled the blood on the doorposts. This should make us all stop and think. Are we living in light, or are we living in darkness? Look around your household. If we have left our families in Egypt, there is not a house where someone is not spiritually dead. Food has not saved us. There are great devastation and nothing green in our lives from what the locusts have eaten. These Scriptures were written as symbols to show us that God is working today in each life so that we can have our own private exodus. God wants us to realize from all the pain that the love of food is worthless and eventually will lead to death of a relationship with Him. But transferring over to God the same attention and heart you have given food is salvation. It is the path to an actual relationship with God. You can be saved from slavery to anything, and God saved the Israelites that very night.

COMPLETE DELIVERANCE

During the night Pharaoh summoned Moses and Aaron and said, "Up! Leave my people, you and the Israelites! Go, worship the LORD as you have requested." . . . At the end of the 430 years, to the very day, all the LORD's divisions left Egypt. . . . By day the LORD went ahead of them in a pillar of cloud to guide them on their way and by night in a pillar of fire to give them light, so that they could travel by day or night. . . . The pillar of cloud also moved from in front and stood behind them, coming between the armies of Egypt and Israel.

Throughout the night the cloud brought darkness to the one side and light to the other side; so neither went near the other all night long. Then Moses stretched out his hand over the sea, and all that night the LORD drove the sea back with a strong east wind and turned it into dry land. The waters were divided, and the Israelites went through the sea on dry ground, with a wall of water on their right and on their left. The Egyptians pursued them, and all Pharaoh's horses and chariots and horsemen followed them into the sea. . . . Then the LORD said to Moses, "Stretch out your hand over the sea so that the waters may flow back over the Egyptians and their chariots and horsemen." (Ex. 12:31, 41; 13:21; 14:19b–23, 26)

At daybreak, the water flowed back and covered the Egyptians. Not one of them survived. Never has there been such complete deliverance!

We have all been enslaved by the world and have looked to the world to save us. But the world is not going to save us from loving it. In fact, the world's remedies are merely disguised incubators that cultivate more love for itself. God has not abandoned us. We have abandoned Him, and we have become distracted and enticed by the glimmer of Egypt, His competitor. But God is a genius as well as the passionate pursuer of our hearts. He knows that we make heroes out of heavyweight champions, that we will follow the winning quarterbacks, that we will throw confetti on the five-star general who strategically wins the battle, and that we will ride away anywhere with the knight in shining armor. God will never allow fat grams to be our Savior or exercise to be our Savior or diet pills to be our Savior. He is our Savior—He has saved us from having to love food, and we get to love Him. He has saved us from having to love the medicine

The world is not going to save us from loving it. In fact, the world's remedies are merely disguised incubators that cultivate more love for itself.

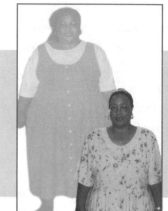

cabinet or the alcohol or the cigarettes, and we get to love Him.

Over the past year, I have lost 87 pounds and am continuing to lose. I am so impressed that God used food to draw me closer to Him and to change my life. When problems arise, I let the heavenly Father solve them instead of a quick fix with food. I am not yet out of the desert, but through obedience to God, I will cross the Jordan.
Hazel James—Cincinnati, OH

Hazel James lost 87 pounds and is drawing closer to God.

So the point has been made—Egypt and Pharaoh were no match for God. On the tenth and final round, Satan and all the world could see that God and God alone was the One to worship, and Egypt was exposed for what it was—worthless and barren. Egypt, after all, could not save itself and could offer no comfort—it wasn't a god after all.

The blood on the doorpost was symbolic of the blood of Christ, and the blood of Christ was never intended to be used to leave us in Egypt with a crush on food. The point of the Passover plague is to spare us and at the same time to catapult us out of Egypt—to drive us out completely and to rescue us entirely!

Besides the Exodus—the great boxing match of all time—God sent Jesus to die for us. He died so that we could have a relationship with God. Jesus' sacrifice opened the door to the heart of God. What have we been doing with this opportunity? What have we been thinking? Don't we realize that even having a chance to be in the presence of God is the ultimate privilege, much less to be *invited* through Jesus Christ to have an intimate relationship with God the Father and Jesus Christ, His Son?

The blood of Christ was used to part the Red Sea, so that we could simply walk across from Egypt to the arms of God on dry land. Then God closed the sea back up on Egypt, leaving a wide chasm between the love of the earth and the love of God, making it impossible to be in both places at once. May we all wake up! God is shaking the walls of Egypt all around you to loosen its grip on you. Look at Egypt—take a good look around you. The world is worthless!

What did I learn behind the walls of that little counseling office in Memphis years ago? Were we overweight due to the wrong food? No. I learned that the problem was that we were in love with food—deeply in love. And there is only one love that has a stronger magnetic pull than the love of food—and it is the love of God. Cutting the food in half and eating only when you are hungry do not change your devotion. You need to transfer your love to the Savior who deserves your love.

If you have covered your doorposts with the blood of Christ, I pray that you will never, ever find your heart stuck between the mortars of the pyramids. I pray that you will never find your heart sinking deep into the middle of the Red Sea, teetering between the love of food and the love of God. I pray that you will find your heart in the center of the Exodus, following God Almighty out of Egypt.

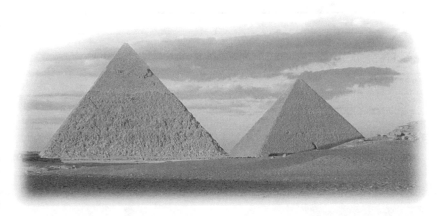

What You Can Do Today

▬▶ *Go where God is leading you in Scripture.*

▬▶ *Put God in first place.* Now that you know that God wants to be your passionate Lover, your Warrior, your five-star General, the Knight who will fight for your honor, and your Hero, what are some changes you can make today that will help you respond to such a King?

▬▶ *Notice the ways God is getting your attention.* Have you endured "plagues" such as tight clothes, shortness of breath, trouble sleeping, and hurtful comments from friends and family? God is simply trying to catapult your heart out of Egypt so that you can enter the desert with Him!

▬▶ *Wake up each day and make the choice to serve the awesome Almighty God instead of the false god of food.* Food can offer you nothing, while the true God can offer you *everything.* Now you can go throughout the rest of your day knowing that you are living to serve a Master who loves you!

_____
_____
_____
_____
_____
_____
_____
_____
_____
_____
_____
_____

Brunches and Buffets

It is always fun to get an invitation from friends to join them for brunch on a weekend or for a special occasion. A brunch usually offers incredible food items such as fresh fruit, scrambled eggs, sausage, bacon, crêpes, waffles, croissants, chicken salad, shrimp cocktail, soups, omelettes, and desserts, and a buffet will offer even more! First and foremost, I invite God into *every* meal because I love Him and I enjoy His food. I worship the Creator instead of the created. Keep your focus on God so that you can love *Him* and not the food. After I invite God into this wonderful eating occasion, I survey all the food choices available at the brunch or buffet. I carefully make my selections based on what flavors and foods I am craving at the time. I take small amounts of the items I want the most, and once I sit down, I even rate the bites within each item, being picky about taking the most sumptuous pieces. As I take a few bites, I sip a non-caloric drink between them, stopping for a moment and putting my utensils down. I look up from the plate and enjoy the company I am with. At a special occasion, such as a bridal or baby shower, I may be sitting with people I am unfamiliar with. Instead of burying my face in my plate, I enjoy some polite conversation or use this time to catch up on what they've been doing lately. I love to be more interested in the company than the food. As a result, I have found that it slows down my eating. And you don't have to do this just at a special function— apply these principles at home with your family. It's a great opportunity to spend time together with your spouse and your children.

four

THE WEIGH DOWN† EXPLOSION

Once I came to understand the fundamental concepts of weight loss and the biblical parallel of the Exodus story, God started stirring the waters. Keep in mind that at this point in the history of Weigh Down†, this information was available only to a few people in a seven-hundred-square-foot counseling office, but these people kept telling me over and over that it was revolutionary, life-transforming information. The number one comment I heard was, "My entire life is changing."

CALLED OUT

One day, after one of my small group lectures, a Weigh Down† participant said, "Look at you, standing here in this retail store, handing out Bibles, and turning people's lives around. This information does not belong in the hands of just a few people. This should be available to everyone!" The comment shocked me. I felt very inadequate because I didn't really know anything about that kind of thing. Then she said, "You already have everything on video and on audio and even in book form. Why don't you let volunteers hold classes and show these videos for you?" My thought was, *Why would anyone want to show these videos?* So at the next meeting, out of curiosity, I explained the concept to the group. Then I passed around a legal pad and asked if people would be willing to show the videos at their church or in a small group setting. Everyone in the room signed up. I was blown away because the people really wanted to help get this idea out. It was the beginning of being *called out*—it certainly wasn't *my* idea or lifelong goal.

I prayed for signs that this was truly the way God would want me to go. Honestly, it scared me to let go of the information. My fear was hard to define. But in three months, by the spring of 1992, I had packaged all the audiocassettes and workbooks, and I expanded the video lessons to include every question that I had ever heard. Immediately, twenty churches signed up, and the program quickly crossed state lines. I could not believe the response. One denomination after another would approve this twelve-week seminar that offered twelve video lessons and twelve audiocassette tapes and a workbook. People willing to work for the company were popping up everywhere—from St. Louis to Birmingham, from Minnesota to Mississippi.

What started in one location in Tennessee spread at the rate of about twenty new churches a month. By January of the following year, new denominations and churches were coming aboard at the rate of sixty per month. Soon the media got wind of this phenomenon, and all at once I found myself doing local newspaper and radio interviews daily. They were all having equal impacts on the growth rate, leading to sixty newly approved classes a week. I really didn't know one magazine, newspaper, or radio show from another, so I thought nothing of it when I got a phone call from *Woman's Day* magazine. The editors were interested in doing a feature on Weigh Down*ᵗ* in an upcoming issue. After prayer, I agreed. God offered another incredible opportunity—I was going to respond to His lead. After I did the interview and gave them some photographs, I wasn't exactly sure when the article would appear or how big it would be.

At that point I had about six in-house employees, plus three outreach directors. When we showed up for work that infamous

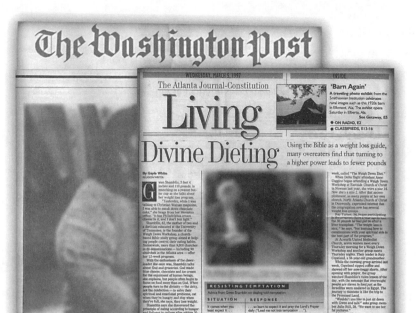

Soon major daily papers were running front-page stories and lifestyle features on the success of Weigh Down†.

Monday in early October, we were not prepared for what was awaiting us. Apparently, all the answering machine cassettes were full, and the phones were ringing off the hooks. We discovered that the *Woman's Day* article had hit the newsstand that weekend with a headline on the cover: "Can God Make You Thin?" Inside the magazine was a four-page article on Weigh Down†. We had four phones with four lines each—we literally answered phones around the clock for nearly two months. As soon as we would press the receiver to end a call, another person would be on the line waiting. During work hours, friends brought us food and we rarely even took bathroom breaks. After hours, we took shifts changing the answering machine cassettes. They filled up at the rate of one per hour. The next morning we would send the cassettes by express service to outreach directors in another city, who would transcribe the information and begin returning calls. We also received massive media requests, faxes, and certified mail. It was a zoo! It was nearly impossible to respond to everyone. This explosion set the pace for the rest of the history of Weigh Down†.

MEDIA ACROSS THE COUNTRY . . . AND THE WORLD

Soon major daily papers like the *New York Times,* the *Washington Post,* the *Houston Chronicle,* the *Miami Herald,* the *Dallas Morning News,* the *Baltimore Sun,* and the *Denver Post* were running front-page stories and lifestyle features about Weigh Down†. Every week we received articles on Weigh Down† torn from papers all across the country. It wasn't long before national publications like *Good Housekeeping, Ladies' Home Journal, U.S. News and World Report, Self, USA Today,* and even the *National Enquirer* (this made my mama proud) took notice and gave significant coverage to the Weigh Down† explosion. My time became consumed with doing media interviews. At that point, there were file cabinets full of newspaper clippings. Nearly every week I was on the radio somewhere in the country—at certain times of the year, it was every day.

The number of Weigh Down† classes mushroomed. After two years we were already in more than five thousand locations. It wasn't long before William Morris, one of the world's largest talent agencies, approached me. The people at the agency were interested in helping me pursue many opportunities, including publishing a book. They introduced me to Doubleday, and *The Weigh Down Diet* was released in March of 1997. That book has sold more than one million copies and remains on the best-seller lists today, by the hand of God only. This book also introduced many to The Weigh Down Workshop† seminars. The William Morris Agency had come to me, and Doubleday had come to me. Once again, I was feeling *called out.* Within months, the number of classes had soared to ten thousand.

The Weigh Down Workshop† caught the attention of some national shows like *Hard Copy* and *A Current Affair* (which featured testimonies of people who had lost at least one hundred pounds or more). Religious programs were delightful, such as *James Robison* and *The 700 Club* with Pat Robertson. Once the seminar classes reached more than 25,000 classes, God was really ready to let the nation know about His great works and phenomenal ability to save people from the desire to overeat. ABC-TV invited me to appear on *The View* and *20/20*. And it wasn't long before I was invited to *Larry King Live* to interview with Larry the entire hour. The interviewers at *The View, 20/20,* and *Larry King Live* all allowed me to speak of God boldly, for they had all seen enough evidence of the power of God and an unprecedented weight loss phenomenon through the video footage we had sent them. They could have eaten me alive, but God somehow closed the mouths of the lions in this medium that rarely credits God. So many people were praying, and God gave me just the right words to answer the tough questions from Larry as well as from the callers. At our office, our phone system temporarily crashed from the call volume (by this time we had more than 60 people capable of answering phones during peak times). The phone company informed us that more than 8,000 people had tried to call at the same instant. Our phones were working again very shortly, and we were able to help thousands of people eager to find out more information. The weekend following the airing of *Larry King Live,* we had 50,000 hits on the Web site. More than 30,000 copies of *The Weigh Down Diet* were sold through retail bookstores within the four weeks following the airing of that show. God was busy, and we were busy. The heart of America was changing before our very eyes—as well as its weight.

The Weigh Down Workshop† has always had an international element. We now have classes in more than 30,000 locations in 70 countries. We have had extensive media coverage throughout Great Britain, Australia, New Zealand, and South Africa, including the *London Observer* and the *London Times,* as well as an inspiring Weigh Down† documentary piece on PBS that aired internationally. God has also blessed the media representation in Canada, Germany, and Sweden. One of the sweetest experiences I can remember was getting to the country of Egypt to refilm the Weigh Down† seminar series and being greeted by two classes of Weigh Downers!

Sometime during this rapid growth phase, it was brought to our attention that there were many Web sites on the Internet created by enthusiastic participants of Weigh Down†. In fact, there were more than 350 of these sites dedicated to Weigh Down†. So we finally caught up with the times and launched an official Weigh Down† Web site in 1997. It already receives nearly a million and a half hits a month by the leading of God. People are discovering The Weigh Down Workshop† and actually joining classes as a result of the Web site. This has also become an incredible tool to expose people in other countries to the Weigh Down† way of life. We receive positive and useful feedback from all over the world and stay in tune with what's happening in the lives of our participants. It's amazing how the Lord is using participants from all around the world to "encourage" one another as the day draws near. The official Weigh Down† Web site address is www.wdworkshop.com. Be sure to look up the testimonial page—it is most inspiring.

In six short years, The Weigh Down Workshop† has grown to a point where it takes more than one hundred employees and many outside consultants and vendors to handle the tasks of this "bursting-at-the-seams" organization. One of our major ministries is an annual convention for coordinators and participants of Weigh Down† called Desert Oasis. Each year, thousands of people from all over the world have attended this wonderful event in Nashville to celebrate what God has done in their lives.

THE GENUINE ARTICLES

It's absolutely remarkable how God has allowed all of this exposure without a single outgoing soliciting phone call from Weigh Down†. We did not pursue this kind of attention or success. It has resulted from God moving people and the news spreading by word of mouth. There are hundreds of thousands of participants—"genuine articles"— who are now free to stop in the middle of a hamburger and have no

Lyn Walker
Franklin, TN
Lost 85 lbs.
Has kept it off
8 years

Anita Pillow
Nashville, TN
Lost 25 lbs.
Has kept it off
6 years

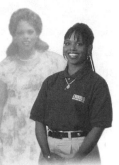

Jeff Venable
Hot Springs, AR
Lost 90 lbs.
Has kept it off
5 years

Debbie Dornfeld
Florissant, MO
Lost 70 lbs.
Has kept it off
6 years

Pam Sneed
St. Peters, MO
Lost 100 lbs.
Has kept it off
4 years

Terry Mangialardi
Olive Branch, MS
Lost 121 lbs.
Has kept it off
5 years

Lee Suddeath
Franklin, TN
Lost 65 lbs.
Has kept it off
6 years

desire to eat the second half. People have called me a genius from time to time, giving me credit for orchestrating all of this. But I am quick to correct them: *God* is the genius. There is no way I could have foreseen what He had in store. In many ways He produced all of this *in spite* of me and my limitations, and it makes me all the more humble, desiring to serve Him and to follow His lead.

Even more impressive than the God-ordained exposure this program has received is to hear the stories of the lives that have been changed by the power of loving Him. The stacks of mail are staggering. Literally truckloads of mail describe the power of God to rescue us from being our own god—in other words, from disastrous, miserable lives! We hear continually from people who have lost from ten to one hundred pounds or more. Also very inspiring are the testimonies from so many ten- to twenty-year-olds who have lost all their extra weight (several in excess of one hundred pounds) and who no longer leave school every day in pain from the snide remarks of their peers. But more important, their eyes light up when they talk about exchanging this relationship with the refrigerator for a close, intimate relationship with Christ. We have seen God's hand continually working in the lives of desperate people. There have been several times that we have received a letter from someone who was getting ready to commit suicide but looked down at the newspaper and saw Weigh Down† being offered at a church or a home setting, then signed up and lost all the extra weight.

People have laid down every kind of stronghold you can imagine, from smoking and alcohol abuse to spending addictions and sexual immorality. The results are unbelievable. No university research center or fat farm can boast the kind of results Weigh Down† has experienced. We are even hearing an outpouring of passionate support from the medical community. They have seen the positive health impact of permanent weight loss as never before! The liquid hospital diets have made many patients sick, but what is worse is that the weight came back after the patients spent $3,000 to $5,000 per session. Because of so many testimonies from doctors, nurses, and others in the medical profession who have lost weight through Weigh Down†, an effort is under way to persuade the medical insurance industry to recognize Weigh Down† participants as eligible for insurance reimbursement of the seminar fee. Also our hope is that the spiritual element of wellness will soon be accepted by corporate health wellness and fitness programs around the country.

It won't be long before this dream is realized. The medical and scientific community is discovering what God revealed to me long ago. A recent report on *NBC Nightly News* heralded the fact that scientists have concluded that "the biggest problem of all is not what you eat; it's how much." Dr. Walter Willett of the Harvard School of Public Health was quoted as saying, "For many years, dietary advice was really based on guesses." The report went on to say that "new studies show the guesses were often wrong. Salt does not usually raise blood pressure. And eggs do not raise cholesterol. The biggest problem of all is not *what* we eat, but *how much* we eat. Whether it is good for you or bad for you, Americans are eating much more of everything—creating an epidemic of obesity."[1] Finally, in 1999, someone else was boldly proclaiming the same thing I had been trying to teach people for years! In the report, Jeanne Goldberg of Tufts University said, "Where we have gone off the deep end is in terms of excess consumption." This is all very encouraging to me— as it should be to you as you journey toward wholehearted devotion to the Father instead of food—but it is discouraging that they are not crediting a program that is pointing people to God and Christ.

People have laid down every kind of stronghold you can imagine.

This massive public response to Weigh Down† was a result of the vacuum of true information. People owned bookcases of diet books, but nothing had ever addressed what to do with the overwhelming desire to binge at ten o'clock at night. No tape or book bridged their spiritual *and* physical needs. Interviewers have always asked, "What does God have to do with weight loss?" Many of them don't seem to get it, but those who struggle with overweight see the connection. The result has been a movement for America—the beginning of the end of dieting and a new hope for permanent thinness. The spiritual impact is immeasurable. So many people have transferred a passion for serving self to serving God. Downcast people have transferred a love for the refrigerator to a love for God and for Jesus Christ.

The Bible tells us, "Likewise every good tree bears good fruit, but a bad tree bears bad fruit. A good tree cannot bear bad fruit, and a bad tree cannot bear good fruit. . . . Thus, by their fruit you will recognize them" (Matt. 7:17–18, 20). Fruit—or results—have always been the way to measure truth, and the results we have seen so far prove that this is a message of truth.

What You Can Do Today

➤ *Go where God is leading you in Scripture.*

➤ *Wait for God to provide for you.* As Weigh Down*t* developed, we did not actively seek media attention or try grabbing anything for ourselves. God provided all the opportunities and placed them at our door. Are you grabbing for honor, praise, or recognition in some situation today? If so, repent and open your life to God, so He can use it in the manner He wishes. He will provide you more fulfilling honor and attention than you could ever grab for yourself. Read James 3:13–18 to learn more about selfish ambition.

➤ *If you have access to the Internet, take a few moments today and read some of the wonderful testimonies on the Weigh Down*t* Web site* (www.wdworkshop.com). Your heart will be touched as you discover how the Father has moved powerfully in the lives of those who are now devoted to *Him* instead of food.

➤ *Consider the fruit.* The Bible tells us that we will recognize "good" and "bad" by the fruit. Think about your old diet plans and programs. Did they yield any permanent fruit in your life or in the lives of people around you? Did they do anything to strengthen your relationship with the Creator? Before you make a decision to devote your time and attention to *anything,* take a moment to consider what fruit it will bear.

_____

_____

_____

_____

_____

_____

Meat Loaf, Mashed Potatoes, and Green Beans

Although I am a working mother, I enjoy preparing an evening meal for my family. When I make meat loaf, I always serve mashed potatoes and green beans with it because this combination has been passed down from generation to generation as a southern tradition. The green beans cooked with ham or bacon create a perfect salt combination—and they bring out the zest in the meat loaf. The meat loaf is prepared with a sweet red tomato sauce, onions, and bell peppers. The combination in the meat loaf alone is enough to savor! The blend of flavors from the onion and the bell pepper seems to enhance the sweet flavor from the red tomato sauce. Not only that, but there are varying textures as well from the ingredients in the meat loaf. Then I love the addition of creamy mashed potatoes. I mash the potatoes with just the right amount of salt, pepper, milk, and butter until they are very creamy. When I add the salty green beans along with the creamy mashed potatoes and zesty meat loaf, I have one of my favorite meal combinations of tastes and textures. To enhance my enjoyment of the meal, I will take several sips of my beverage or a taste of a dinner roll between bites. I find that this washes the taste of the green beans from my palate so that I can fully enjoy the flavor of the meat loaf. Sometimes, I even take a small portion from every grouping of tastes and textures to create one special bite! Most important, I praise God for each bite, I eat slowly, and I eat only *small portions*—very small. Three peanut M&Ms top off the meal, and my mind is free from food until my stomach growls again. Praise God!

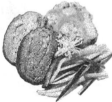

five

THE STRUGGLER

Please do not feel bad if you have struggled. We live in a world that bombards us with a massive amount of information, and it is easy to get sidetracked. You may have lost one hundred pounds and gained some, or even all, of it back. You may have joined a Weigh Down† seminar and never quite got the hang of it. You may have lost your weight but are still battling temptations frequently. Don't worry about all of that. I want you to know that God has put in my heart a love for each of you, and I truly wish I could give every one of you a hug and a sweet word of encouragement.

You are truly a precious eternal creation who has been given a world of choices. I understand that there is much confusion, but do not give up. I'm telling you—you can't give up now. You're going to make it. The victory is going to be sweet and worth the searching and the battles. God is the God of all comfort, and we are weary sojourners. If you are needing more comfort right now, please be sure to refer to chapter 9, "Save Your Heart for Me." Remember that your weight problem has caused you to cry out to God, and it is bringing you closer to God. You will eventually appreciate the thing that has caused you so much pain, for it will bring you into a deep and permanent relationship with the God of the universe.

Weigh Down† has been available in churches since 1992 and is becoming very well known. As a result, there have been numerous "copycats" and many tempting diet plans to run to when the going gets tough. I know that eating less food is going to be the most difficult battle that some of you will ever face in your lifetime. You were brought up to clean your plate and to worship and focus wholeheartedly on food. This chapter is going to discuss many of the tempting diet plans and arguments against The Weigh Down Workshop[†]. I hope you will see more clearly the logic and the reason for eating God's way.

It Is Not Wrong to Defend the Truth

There will always be Satan-inspired differences, even by people who claim to be followers of Christ. God allows for false teachers so that we will be prompted to dig and seek for *truth*. He doesn't just hand truth to us on a silver platter. Divisions and differences are going to happen when two forces are out there—good and evil. But following a false teacher is wrong, and we will be responsible and accountable to God for supporting wrong teachers and false teachings. Jesus said there will be five in a household, three against two and two against three (Luke 12:52). He also said that He did not come to bring peace, but a sword (Matt. 10:34). Hebrews 4:12–13 says, "For the word of God is living and active. Sharper than any double-edged sword, it penetrates even to dividing soul and spirit, joints and marrow; it judges the thoughts and attitudes of the heart. Nothing in all creation is hidden from God's sight. Everything is uncovered and laid bare before the eyes of him to whom we must give account."

There is nothing wrong with arguments. God allows for debates. The Apostle Paul debated the Jewish Sanhedrin court and the Pharisees, who were the religious leaders of the day (Acts 22:30–23:10). Jesus was constantly debating and reasoning with the Pharisees. Jesus even ran money-grubbers out of the temple court areas (Matt. 21:12). God Himself says in Scripture: "Come now, let

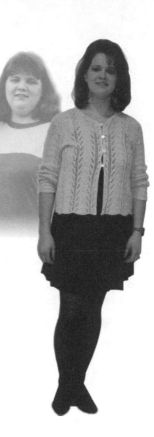

I lost 30 pounds the very first session of Weigh Down†, but then I entered the desert. I alternated from being very obedient to being halfhearted and then downright rebellious. One day I was reminded by a friend that I was willfully sinning by overeating and not feeling sorry for it, and therefore hardened by sin's deceitfulness. The next morning I opened my Bible to Hebrews 3:7–8: "Today, if you hear his voice, do not harden your hearts as you did in the rebellion." This was exactly what I was doing! I lay there repenting and begging God to forgive me. I have lost 90 pounds so far, and I have found glorious freedom in Jesus and in the security of a Father who will discipline me when He has to. What an awesome God we serve!

Danette Bishop—Nampa, ID
Lost 90 lbs.

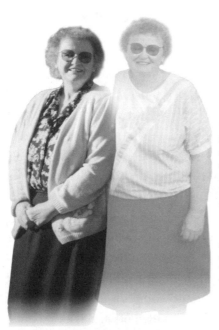

Through Weigh Down†, the Lord started dealing with my heart. I never realized how strong and powerful my will was. I went through struggle after struggle—I'd do it the Lord's way, then slip back into my way. I was finally convinced that His way was the best and only way. For the first time in my life, I have the hope of being a thin eater for the rest of my life! I have lost 55 pounds, my daughter has lost 50 pounds, and our family has been set free from generations of bondage to food. Praise God!
Marion Wells—Lynchburg, VA
Lost 55 lbs.

us reason together" (Isa. 1:18a). So come along with me and let's reason together using God's Word, so that you can be assured that you are following God's truth—not Gwen's or anyone else's.

DIETS, RAW FOOD PLANS, AND BIOLOGICAL FEEDBACK

New programs that have been popping up over the last few years are agreeing with bits and pieces of Weigh Down†, but they are not endorsing the major concepts. In other words, they may agree with the hunger and fullness concept, but then they tell you that you can eat only certain foods. Then there are those programs that suggest it is too hard to find hunger and fullness—they don't even know what hunger and fullness are. They make suggestions that we are to eat only raw foods or uncooked foods and, on top of that, claim to back up the suggestion with Scripture. There are others that insist they know exactly what the human should consume. They imply that the body does not have a biological feedback mechanism, and that, indeed, you would be sick if you ate what your body craved.

Projection Is Common, but Wrong

You've got to keep in mind that when you have struggled or failed with The Weigh Down Workshop†, the hardest thing in the world to do is to admit that you have not eaten less food. The human was made with a strong self-preservation instinct, and it will rarely point a finger at itself first. Keep in mind that Cain killed his own brother (Gen. 4:8) because (1) Cain felt that Abel made him look bad, and (2) if Cain could put down or get rid of the source of truth, it would allow him to do whatever he wanted to do—or so he thought. Poor reasoning. Cain would have been better off to let Abel live and just continually try to imitate Abel's behavior until he got it right. God is patient with that attitude only up to a point. But if you look at history, mankind has always killed off and tried to quiet the prophets who were asking *them,* rather than the environment around them, to change.

God has blessed The Weigh Down Workshop†, and many people have been through the program. And some have not lost all their weight. But if you stumble, be very careful that you do not try to lay blame on the people around you or on the situation. And be careful that you do not make the mistake of grabbing hold of a program that wants the food to change. I know how hard it is to change your own heart. If I hadn't gone through it myself, how could I have written this book? It can be very hard, and there are times when I would rather have died first. But I promise you that good health, longevity, and a healthy spiritual relationship come from focusing on reading the labels on your own heart, studying the content of your heart, stirring up a new recipe in your heart, and finally, boiling off the self-indulgence in your own heart by obeying God's Word (1 Peter 1:22).

You've got to keep in mind that when you have struggled or failed with The Weigh Down Workshop†, the hardest thing in the world to do is to admit that you have not eaten less food.

What About Levitical Food Laws?

All the counterarguments to The Weigh Down Workshop† are similar in that they try to undermine the truths that God *can* direct each person on "what" and "how much" to eat and that there *is* an internal control or a guidance from God. We should believe that God has a genius design that tells us when we are hungry and when we are full, as well as what to eat (see the section on biological feedback in this chapter). Each of the counterarguments tries to make you believe that there are good foods and bad foods, and that "its program" happens to have the list of foods that God wants you to swallow. Some will even take Scriptures out of context and suggest that you follow the Old Testament Levitical laws with food. If we are to follow the Levitical laws, or even laws that predate Moses, with regard to food rules, then where do we draw the line? Are we to follow *all* the rules? A quick review of the Levitical laws lets us know that these rules include all kinds of purification and animal sacrifices and detailed out-of-the-camp rules for infectious diseases and mildew (Lev. 1–27; Num. 15; 18; 19; Deut. 14–26). Following these laws is tough; for example, "If anyone curses his father or mother, he must be put to death. . . . If a man commits adultery with another man's wife—with the wife of his neighbor—both the adulterer and the adulteress must be put to death" (Lev. 20:9–10). Keep in mind that the Apostle Paul warned in Galatians 5:1–4,

It is for freedom that Christ has set us free. Stand firm, then, and do not let yourselves be burdened again by a yoke of slavery. Mark my words! I, Paul, tell you that if you let yourselves be circumcised [a law that predated Moses and also a law of Moses], Christ will be of no value to you at all. Again I declare to every man who lets himself be circumcised that he is obligated to obey the whole law. You who are trying to be justified by law have been alienated from Christ; you have fallen away from grace.

The New Testament clearly points out that we do not have to follow the food rules of the Old Testament. First of all, Jesus pronounced *all* foods "clean" in Mark 7:19. The meaning here is that Jesus got rid of the "clean" and "unclean" food rules. There were only a few food laws and Levitical laws that we have to carry over into the new covenant. In a letter to the early Christians, the apostles and elders in Jerusalem wrote, "It seemed good to the Holy Spirit and to us not to burden you with anything beyond the following requirements: You are to abstain from foods sacrificed to idols, from blood, from the meat of strangled animals and from sexual immorality. You will do well to avoid these things" (Acts 15:28–29). First Corinthians 10:25–26 tells us, "Eat anything sold in the meat market without raising questions of conscience, for, 'The earth is the Lord's, and every-thing in it.'" In general, Christians are not to follow the Levitical food laws or push them on anyone. Notice how the Apostle Paul reacted when even the Apostle Peter, who did miraculous signs, tried to force Jewish customs:

> *When Peter came to Antioch, I opposed him to his face, because he was clearly in the wrong. Before certain men came from James, he used to eat with the Gentiles. But when they arrived, he began to draw back and separate himself from the Gentiles because he was afraid of those who belonged to the circumcision group. The other Jews joined him in his hypocrisy, so that by their hypocrisy even Barnabas was led astray. When I saw that they were not acting in line with the truth of the gospel, I said to Peter in front of them all, "You are a Jew, yet you live like a Gentile and not like a Jew. How is it, then, that you force Gentiles to follow Jewish customs? We who are Jews by birth and not 'Gentile sinners' know that a man is not justified by observing the law, but by faith in Jesus Christ. So we, too, have put our faith in Christ Jesus that we may be justified by faith in Christ and not by observing the law, because by observing the law no one will be justi-fied." (Gal. 2:11–16)*

What About Food Plans That Suggest Only Raw Foods?

I have noticed that people who claim that we are to eat only raw fruits or vegetables do not use the entire Bible but use only *one* verse in the Bible: "Then God said, 'I give you every seed-bearing plant on the face of the whole earth and every tree that has fruit with seed in it. They will be yours for food'" (Gen. 1:29). This verse was the rule for man in Paradise, but after the great Flood, God instructed us, "Everything that lives and moves will be food for you. Just as I gave you the green plants, I now give you *everything*. But you must not eat meat that has its lifeblood still in it" (Gen. 9:3–4, italics added). We must be careful not to take Scripture out of context. How could you possibly know God's way if you do not read past the first chapter of Genesis?

God's Word, taken as a whole, does not back up programs that encourage eating only *raw* foods. In fact, God Himself provided His children with food to be cooked. When the Israelites were wandering in the desert after being delivered from slavery in Egypt, God provided them with manna to eat. It was a form of bread that miraculously appeared with the morning dew (Num. 11:9). The manna was gathered every morning, except on the Sabbath (Ex. 16:26). The Israelites prepared the manna various ways. After gathering their share for the day, they "ground it in a handmill or crushed it in a mortar. They cooked it in a pot or made it into cakes. And it tasted like something made with olive oil" (Num. 11:8). Exodus 16:23b notes that when talking about the manna, the Lord commanded the Israelites, "Bake what you want to bake and boil what you want to boil."

Keep in mind that if you don't cook certain foods—such as meat or eggs—you are swallowing loads of bacteria, amoebas, and microbes. Prepare to be sick on a strict raw food diet for the following reasons: first, consumption of only raw vegetables and fruits is *not* what your body craves, and you will surely be missing some nutrients. You will discover after a few days of eating just raw vegetables and fruits that you desire to eat bread (cooked grains), meats, cheese, or milk. By the way, cheese and milk are processed foods. "Processed" means that the food has been handled in some way. Even an apple has had human hands on it. It is plucked from the tree and often washed (processed). Most apples are sprayed with a harmless wax to keep them from dehydrating before they get to the consumer. The wax protects the consumer from bacteria and other harmful substances that could enter the skin of the apple. No one promoted the "processing" of foods more than God Himself (see the section on processed foods later in this chapter). Therefore, processing foods is not against God's will.

The Israelites were told to go to extraordinary measures to make sure that the food was clean and protected! Leviticus 11:31b–35, 37–38 states:

> *Whoever touches them* [unclean animals] *when they are dead will be unclean till evening. When one of them dies and falls on something, that article, whatever its use, will be unclean, whether it is made of wood, cloth, hide or sackcloth. Put it in water; it will be unclean till evening, and then it will be clean. If one of them falls into a clay pot, everything in it will be unclean, and you must break the pot. Any food that could be eaten but has water on it from such a pot is unclean, and any liquid that could be drunk from it is unclean. Anything that one of their carcasses falls on becomes unclean; an oven or cooking pot must be broken up. They are unclean, and you are to regard them as unclean. . . . If a carcass falls on any seeds that are to be planted, they remain clean. But if water has been put on the seed and a carcass falls on it, it is unclean for you.*

A second reason you should prepare to get sick if you eat only raw or uncooked foods is that you will develop a spastic colon and have painful gas. This is the body's way (biological feedback) of telling you to stop doing this. On the other hand, people who eat what the body is craving will experience an improvement in digestion.

Biological Feedback

First of all, some people do not believe the Weigh Down† teaching that there is biological feedback or that there is a dependable feedback mechanism, so they think you must follow food rules. Never mind that all—*all*—the animals know exactly what to eat! Each species eats the same things. They are geniuses, huh? Why do we question this instinct in mankind? Have we *no* instincts programmed by God? But think again. Do you measure the amount of oxygen your body needs? Do you not instinctively walk out of a room filled with smoke because it bothers you? You breathe deeply when you finally get out into fresh air. Your body will cause you to sneeze when you breathe air filled with car fumes or even too much perfume. The amount of oxygen you need is directly proportional (one-to-one ratio) to the amount of glucose (broken-down food) you require, as illustrated in the Krebs cycle. Why would God give you the ability to measure the exact oxygen you need but not the glucose?

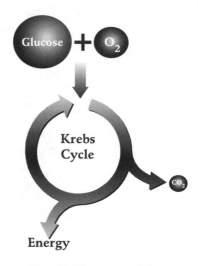

You can tell how many calories you need by measuring your oxygen intake since they are needed in equal amounts.

Think about it—do you control your hormones for monthly cycles, puberty, pregnancy, or even adrenaline releases when you are fearful? Can you not sense an adrenaline release in your body? Well, then, how about a hydrochloric acid release in the stomach for hunger? Do we not see God's involvement in conception? Read Genesis 30. Genesis 30:22–23a states, "Then God remembered Rachel; he listened to her and opened her womb. She became pregnant and gave birth to a son." God gives the animals sleep cycles. Some are nocturnal and some are not. Who teaches the animals this? God is not limited in how He can guide us. He uses full-grown adult animals to teach the young animals how to gather the food for which they are instinctively hungry. Likewise, we pass down learned eating habits to our own children. Some are good and some are bad. Any greedy, godless habits are not good.

There has been some discussion by various people that you would be sick or unhealthy if you ate what your body "wanted." Another way to say this is, "I couldn't possibly be healthy if I just ate what I *wanted.*" The people who make these arguments have obviously not read the entire *Weigh Down Diet* or participated in a Weigh Down† seminar. What Weigh Down† teaches is that there is a God-given bio-logical feedback. This feedback in its pure form will "want" a variety. If you are eating the volume your body calls for and listening to "what" your body calls for, your eating will be balanced. If you are greedy for chocolate or "want" only chocolate for days and days, you will need to be still and pray before you eat. Just as you have to sub-due the "want" to overeat and follow your body's cues, you need to be obedient to your body's natural desire for variety.

In a society that has grown up under "no-no" foods and diets—that is, heavy restrictions—there have been isolated instances reported where people have binged out on certain foods once they were freed up. This is sometimes a necessary part of the journey toward freedom because you find out that you become sick of the food that you *think* you can't stop eating. This is biological feedback. Biological feedback can come in many forms and fashions. But just as hunger and fullness are real feelings that can be ignored, you can ignore the God-given food choice of biological feedback. For example, some people ignore the biological feedback that the body gives when they eat too much sugar—the spastic colon or diarrhea, the stomach-aches, and the repulsion sensation felt high up in the esophagus. Some people even ignore their teeth rotting out! But this is biologi-cal feedback in its last stages. Please learn to listen to your body.

One exercise I always suggest when someone starts in a Weigh Down† seminar class is the *chocolate (or your favorite binge food) test.* This exercise will convince you that there *is* biological feedback. In other words, it will show you that your body *can* tell you that you have had enough. Many people believe if they gave themselves the freedom to eat anything, they would binge out on chocolate or chips and dip till the grave. This is not true. If you have a binge food—chocolate, for example—just try eating *only chocolate* for an entire day. Eat chocolate for breakfast while everyone else at the table is having bacon and bagels or eggs and toast. Eat chocolate for lunch while your coworkers are eating hamburgers fixed with mustard, lettuce, onion, and tomatoes, along with French fries with ketchup and salt, and a diet soda. Then, eat chocolate for your afternoon snack while everyone else is enjoying salty buttered popcorn. Finally, eat chocolate for supper while the family enjoys meat loaf, creamed potatoes with butter and salt and pepper, green beans, yeast rolls, and iced tea with lemon. You will feel sick after the first twelve hours. If not then, soon after. Let me assure you that there *is* biofeedback—*strong* biofeedback—and you must believe this. Learn about it and wake it up! You have been burying it under rule books and sheets of paper telling you what to do.

When you get your volume in line with the will of God through His hunger and fullness, then you can fine-tune your nutritional status by learning to be still and to listen to what your body is calling for. I do not believe that you can make many mistakes here because *Variety ensures you the nutrients you need—that is why God did not give Adam and Eve a food pyramid list.* the body has such a strong drive to get a variety of foods. Even the most "out of touch to what the body wants" people will not eat what they had for breakfast again for lunch and what they had for lunch again for supper and will complain when leftovers are offered. In other words, they are in touch with the body's biological feedback enough to eat a variety even within a twenty-four-hour period. This guarantees a spectrum of nutrients because your body cues you to an assortment of foods. Variety ensures you the nutrients you need—that is why God did not give Adam and Eve a food pyramid list. He programs guidance inside His children, and when a person submits to this natural guidance, he will not overeat and will be well nourished. Not only does God program what you need inside you; He programs your taste buds to like it, and He provides your body with the enzymes to digest it.

It is all delightfully simple and enjoyable if we get the will out of the way. Keep in mind that Scripture points out another whole category of health measures that we human beings should take if we desire optimum health. This is pointed out in *The Weigh Down Diet* and in Scripture. For example, Proverbs 4:20–22 states,

> *My son, pay attention to what I say;*
> *listen closely to my words.*
> *Do not let them out of your sight,*
> *keep them within your heart;*
> *for they are life to those who find them*
> *and health to a man's whole body.*

I can testify that keeping God's words in my heart and applying them to my life and being obedient to His Word have given me sweet sleep and a healthy body. Proverbs 3:7–8 tells us,

> *Do not be wise in your own eyes;*
> *fear the* LORD *and shun evil.*
> This *will bring health to your body*
> *and nourishment to your bones.* (emphasis added)

When you realize that the eternal part of your being—your mind, heart, and spirit—is a big part of your being, it is easy to understand how getting your mind and heart and spirit right will affect your entire health. Haven't you seen people full of hate who become almost physically affected and prematurely aged from it? I have. And on the other hand, there are older people I know who are full of the Spirit of God. Their eyes shine and they are bubbly, energetic, happy, and hopeful. I beg of you to be obedient to God.

What About Processed Foods?

And what about processed foods? Where did we get the idea that processing foods was evil or dangerous or not of God? We need to think things through and realize that man-made rules are everywhere, and we need to stay in God's Word so that we can be wary of the man-made rules and be informed of God's rules. God asks us to process foods: get them cleaned up, cook them, mix ingredients together, and so on. We think, *The Bible must be obsolete because they didn't have processed foods back then.* But think again. Take a look at Leviticus and the offerings that were ordained by God and prepared and eaten in that time. They ate their tithe . . .

> *If you bring a grain offering baked in an oven, it is to consist of fine flour: cakes made without yeast and mixed with oil, or wafers made without yeast and spread with oil. If your grain offering is prepared on a griddle, it is to be made of fine flour mixed with oil, and without yeast. Crumble it and pour oil on it; it is a grain offering. . . . Every grain offering you bring to the LORD must be made without yeast, for you are not to burn any yeast or honey in an offering made to the LORD by fire. You may bring them to the LORD as an offering of the firstfruits, but they are not to be offered on the altar as a pleasing aroma. Season all your grain offerings with salt. Do not leave the salt of the covenant of your God out of your grain offerings; add salt to all your offerings.* (Lev. 2:4–6, 11–13)

Processed fine flour, spread with oil and salt—my, that grain offering is very similar to our richest and saltiest chips! Notice that God asked them to use "fine" flour. Keep in mind that these instructions were given sometime around 1500 B.C. These people had to take grain from the field, thresh it to separate the wheat from the chaff, and then grind this grain mixture down into the finest of flours. Remember, *God* asked for this. We just don't know Him as we ought to. Get to know Him, and you will love Him for letting you enjoy what He has already programmed inside you. We just need to get our own evil desires for extra food out of the way, and we know when we have had too many sweets or too much to drink that we should not have. The Spirit of God within you is "self-control." The only evil associated with eating is worshiping the food and becoming greedy with it. Don't love the food and enjoy God—love God *first,* and enjoy His food!

The New Testament gives us many examples of the freedom in eating. For instance, Jesus drank wine, and the prodigal son was offered red meat. The Bible diets had virtually nothing of the basic four food groups or the new food pyramid groups taught today.

Contrary to popular opinion, fats are not evil. God made fats to create flavor in foods. And the fat content of food creates its aroma. Without smell, you could not taste flavor. Fats enhance the smell because the flavor of the food is trapped into the fat molecules. That is why you can smell bacon cooking, but not oatmeal. So fats enhance your enjoyment of the flavor of food. Fats make foods more appealing and easier to swallow. Fats will float to the top of your stomach in a meal and make you feel sated or full. If you eat only raw vegetables and fruits, you will constantly be hungry, never feeling this full feeling. And this will just make you constantly focused on foods. Eat a regular meal, and then you can move on to other things in this life. There is so much to do and so much to see and so much more living to do than fooling with and thinking about food all day.

Look at this passage: "From what he offers he is to make this offering to the LORD by fire: all the fat that covers the inner parts or is connected to them, both kidneys with the fat on them near the loins, and the covering of the liver, which he will remove with the kidneys. The priest shall burn them on the altar as food, an offering made by fire, a pleasing aroma. All the fat is the LORD's" (Lev. 3:14–16). God would not have asked for the fat portions if there was something wrong with them. And He refers to the pleasing aroma. The truth is that fats are vital to proper bodily functions, including healthy nails and hair. Too much fat is not good for you, but too much vitamin A is not good for you, either. It is toxic in large quantities and can kill you. *Moderation* is the key, and it allows you to eat anything—even fats and sweets.

And What About Preservatives, Food Additives, and Toxic Substances?

To start with, there are very dependable agencies that monitor our food supply. The CDC (Centers for Disease Control) is responsible for many things, including food-borne diseases. The EPA (Environmental Protection Agency) regulates pesticides and establishes water quality standards. You have probably heard of the FAO (Food and Agriculture Organization), the FDA (Food and Drug Administration), and the USDA (United States Department of Agriculture), which are responsible for ensuring the safety and wholesomeness of all foods sold in interstate commerce. These agencies inspect food plants and imported foods, and they set standards for food composition. All of these agencies regulate food industries and help educate the population.

Consumers who have not had a chemistry class are surprised to find out that *all* foods are made up of chemicals and that their own bodies are even made up of chemicals. We would be naive to think that we could eliminate chemicals from our diet. We would have nothing to eat. There are natural toxicants everywhere. The possibility that harmful substances might be contaminating our food is very small because the FDA regulates this, and unsafe amounts are removed from the market. The U.S. government has what it calls the GRAS (Generally Recognized As Safe) list of foods. This list is established by the Congress of the United States to cover substances added to food. The government operates under the strictest laws to make sure that a food contains no carcinogens (cancer-causing agents). These laws state that "no additive shall be deemed to be safe if it is found to induce cancer when ingested (at any level) by man or animal." Today, scientific understanding of cancer has progressed, and technology has advanced to the point that carcinogens in foods can be detected even when they are present in a few parts per trillion.

We have bought into the food phobias, and again, this causes us to focus on the food. These phobias are exacerbated by entrepreneurs who want to sell you their "clean" product. Those are the foods, I promise you, that I am scared to eat! Often these foods—such as processed barley products—are marketed as "health supplements" in order to bypass FDA monitoring and regulation, and they are often sold by individuals in direct pyramid sales. And don't be fooled by the label "all natural." Substances in their unprocessed, natural state can actually be quite toxic. *Be careful!*

Why are there so many reported cases of cancer nowadays if the food is inspected? Well, first of all, we are all going to die, and God takes us out one way or another. We do not have shorter life spans in this decade—in fact, they are longer. Our foods are the same or better than they were one hundred years ago, but not worse. We didn't keep accurate records many years ago. The death certificate likely read, "Old Man Joseph died in his sleep on February 1, 1869." He could have died from cancer. Why are we letting ourselves be convinced that things are worse today? We need to be concentrating on the condition of our depleted hearts, not the depleted soil. One is eternal, and one is temporal.

Why Do We Love Diets?

Why do we want to cling to having food rules? Well, for one thing, we want to stay as close to our idol as we can. Lust is a fleshly feeling that we want to have—and yet it is a counterfeit feeling that leaves us empty and wanting more. We may not get to eat everything we like on these diets, but at least the diet allows us to dream about it. But if you follow a misguided teacher who discusses foods, asks you to read the labels and examine the foods, endorses special preparations, and gives you a new food rule to adhere to every week, then that misguided leader is encouraging you to lust after your idol instead of turning you away from it.

I have warned you from the beginning. I have pleaded with you to stop dieting and to stop these "special foods" programs because if you are lusting after food all day long, you cannot stop overeating. You will *never* lose the weight. God's rule is to stop being greedy. There is no way to stop the lust if you are told to focus on and prepare certain special categories of foods. The only way to stop lusting is to not think about food until you are hungry and then get what you are craving. That is *moderation* and appropriate enjoyment of foods. Not too little and not too much.

Why do we want to cling to having food rules? Well, for one thing, we want to stay as close to our idol as we can.

What if your problem was pornography and you joined a program that told you not to indulge in these graphic movies anymore? Imagine if the method (or program) gave everyone pictures of people half-dressed (the equivalent of our low-calorie foods). They would then meet in support groups to share the new, half-dressed pictures. The group could even exchange these new, halfway cleaned-up pictures with each other. With this focus, who would be set free from lusting and desiring for more?

Remember what I said earlier about the alcoholic. What if a support group leader suggested that every alcoholic in the support group just drink low-alcohol beverages, share favorite low-alcohol recipes, sample each other's concoctions, look at pictures of mixed drinks, examine all the ingredients in each beverage, and talk about alcohol in every meeting? Do you think that that person would ever be free from the lust for alcohol? The answer is, "Of course not."

It is amazing, but many of us might prefer to be with, lust over, and talk about *food* rather than the *Creator of food*. But when we realize this and face this truth, then we *can* escape. We can get it straight. Please escape. Do not focus on foods or their contents. Do not worry about the content of the food; instead, worry about your eternal heart, and examine your motives for wanting to diet, read food rules, follow Jewish customs, resurrect the food laws for Adam and Eve (raw foods), or pick Noah's food rules. Please do not pick and choose from Old Testament food rules that have been set down by Jesus (Mark 7) and the apostles (Acts 15). Do you know more than God's great men who wrote the New Testament Scriptures?

DIET PILLS

What about diet pills? Well, at least these pills don't encourage you to examine and focus on foods, but these "helps" or "counterfeit" appetite suppressants will not help your heart to desire less food, and they do not help with the speed of weight loss. You cannot beat the speed of weight loss that is found in a Weigh Down† participant who understands. However, people naively think they can lose weight "more quickly" or "more easily" by taking pills.

Diuretics can temporarily make you lose some water weight, but they never remove fat, and they are damaging to your kidneys. Obesity does not cause water retention. In fact, obese people have a smaller percentage of body water than their normal-weight counterparts. Therefore, the obese person is in more danger of dehydrating. Loss of water weight is extremely temporary. The number on the scales may have changed for a few hours, but when you consume water the next day, the number on the scales goes right back up.

Amphetamines are "uppers," and the dizziness, nausea, diarrhea, blurred vision, irritability, and light-headedness are similar to feelings you might have when taking very high doses of caffeine. These pills speed up your heart rate and are damaging to the heart and other organs. The FDA no longer approves amphetamines for weight loss, and by the way, they may curb your appetite for a few minutes, but they do *nothing* to curb your desire eating, head hunger, or greed. In fact, my belief is that they contribute to some of the binge eating cycles that are becoming more of a dominant pattern of the dieter. The only things that curb your greed are humility and fear and obedience to God. (See James 4:4–9.) The appetite that needs to be suppressed is your own desire to indulge yourself more and more and more. This is not the attitude of Jesus Christ. Jesus' food was to "do the will of the Father," and that food gives back to you—but feeding and indulging yourself leave you empty. This is the mystery of the cross of Christ. *This* is the information that you need to be digesting,

not a diuretic, amphetamine, or some neurotransmitter like sero-
tonin that depresses the hunger mechanism temporarily. The true
physical hunger mechanism is hardly a player in obesity. Rather, it's
this monstrous head hunger that we need to suppress and this deep-
seated spiritual hunger that we need to learn how to satisfy. The
next few chapters are strategic because they will accomplish both.

DESPERATE MEASURES

I am very aware of how desperate Americans are to lose weight and
how much of a need there is to reroute this passion that many people
have for the refrigerator. Surgical methods such as doing gastric bypass procedures, cutting off the fat, sucking the fat out with suction-
assisted lipectomies, putting balloons in the stomach, and wiring the
jaw are extremely drastic measures used by hopeless and hurting
people. The irony is that *none* of these major, painful, dangerous, and
life-threatening measures address the soul's craving for more food
and for comfort and for love. Therefore, they do *nothing* to help eliminate gaining all the weight back after spending so much money and
energy and sacrificing your health.

Let's look at one area in particular: gastric bypass surgeries. You
know that something is wrong when we start having to completely
reroute the food from the way God has planned it. A
bypass operation implies that you are bypassing the small
intestines, which is where all foods are broken down
and absorbed. Someone undergoing this procedure
will experience severe malnutrition within several months, and if she wants to live, she will
eventually need to reconnect the digestive
tract the way God made it. The result is that
the patient inevitably regains her weight, yet
overall may have done severe damage to the
health of the body as a whole.

Creating a shortcut in your digestive system will not remove the greed in your heart for more food.

One of my major concerns is that very few of the proponents of gastric bypasses (and the only ones I have ever seen promote this procedure are those who are profiting from it) discuss the severe pain that results from a lack of having any normal digestion. Undigested and partially digested and absorbed foods are being routed from the stomach to the lower colon too quickly, causing the "dumping syndrome" symptoms of nausea, weakness, sweating, faintness, and diarrhea after eating. Bypassing God's naturally designed digestive route will leave you in a lot of pain and depression, with an underlying fear and guilt. You will sense that you are not digesting food properly, and you may begin to experience the early signs of malnutrition—your hair starting to fall out and your nails becoming weaker. In fact, because the food moves through your digestive system too quickly for needed nutrients to be absorbed, you will be required to consume large quantities of vitamins and minerals each day in order to avoid becoming malnourished.

People who turn to this drastic surgery are only exacerbating their situation. I have counseled many people who have had a gastric bypass and wish they had known about other alternatives before they made that decision. Not only is gastric bypass surgery very dangerous, but it also has *no value* in helping the *heart* to *desire less food.* In fact, the very words that it boasts are "It allows the person to continue to eat to his heart's desire,

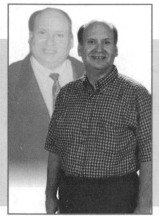

> Since high school I had dieted with the best of them: counting calories, the powdered drink diet, the soup diet, the water diet, diets that required hormone shots, low fat/low sugar diets, and then the ultimate—gastric bypass surgery in 1983. The gastric bypass worked wonders for two years. Then the weight returned with a vengeance. I didn't have enough sense at the time to realize that it wasn't the gastric bypass that was failing me. It was my overeating and stuffing my little stomach pouch way past full. My focus was on the gastric bypass as the answer, not on my heavenly Father.
> **Pastor Dennis Sigle—Burlington, IN—Lost 104 pounds**

After joining Weigh Down† at his church, Dennis Sigle recognized that God, not medical procedures, offered a permanent solution to his overweight condition.

and yet lose weight." So again, this procedure does *nothing* to change the focus of the heart and mind. You need to reroute your *passion,* not your God-designed digestive system.

ANOREXIA, BULIMIA, AND OTHER EATING DISORDERS

In anorexia and bulimia, the person is using his or her own willpower to avoid following God's plan for eating. To start with, the person dealing with anorexia, bulimia, or any eating disorder must realize that obeying God's design of hunger and fullness has *never* made anyone overweight! To the contrary, it keeps people thin. But instead of following God's design, people with eating disorders try to be their own god, using severe bodily deprivation, harsh treatment of the body, and/or excessive exercise to "control" their body size. This is really just another form of dieting. An eating disorder is *not* a disease, and you *are* capable of walking right out of this today.

However, the bottom line is that we are not good gods. We say, "It's *my* body, and I'm going to control it the way I want to control it, and I am not going to be overweight the way my mother was, no matter what it takes." So we come up with our own set of rules, and we work to meet those rules. We justify our actions, we feel pretty good about it, and we feel self-righteous, so to speak (read Rom. 10:1–4). But look at what 1 Corinthians 3:16–17

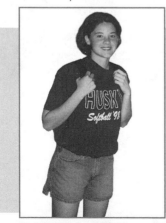

I kept thinking, Eating disorders don't happen to girls like me. *The more I looked at myself, the more disgusted I got. I was totally focused inward on myself. I had heard of other girls at my school who were bulimic. They were skinny, and it looked as if they had it all together. That's when I started throwing up. I would come home, eat dinner, throw it up, and then run two miles. I think God used my eating disorder to open my heart up to Him. From the first day of Weigh Down†, I was ready to change. Now I eat when I'm hungry and stop when I'm full. I don't feel guilty any more, because I know God is in control.*
Jen Jurgensmeyer—Overland Park, KS

God helped Jen Jurgensmeyer to first confront, then overcome, her eating disorder.

says: "Don't you know that you yourselves are God's temple and that God's Spirit lives in you? If anyone destroys God's temple, God will destroy him; for God's temple is sacred, and you are that temple." What the anorexic or bulimic or dieter fails to realize is that contrary to her belief, it is *not* her body! God created it—every system and every cell—and it is *His* temple.

Dieters of any type are the perfect example of "self-disciplined" controllers who have not tasted the fruit of "God-control." People who keep using their own strength to get by are not new. The prophet Isaiah spoke God's words:

> *You were wearied by all your ways,*
>> *but you would not say, "It is hopeless."*
> *You found renewal of your strength,*
>> *and so you did not faint. . . .*
> *I will expose your righteousness and your works,*
>> *and they will not benefit you.*
> *When you cry out for help,*
>> *let your collection of idols save you!* (Isa. 57:10, 12–13a)

People who use their own strength eventually become exhausted. The work of their hands does not bear fruit that will last.

Jesus said, "Come to me, all you who are weary and burdened, and I will give you rest" (Matt. 11:28). Whether it is raw food diets, pills or drugs, gastric bypasses, or throwing up food and taking laxatives and diuretics, God is telling us to *repent* from depending on false helps that change the body without changing the soul. Do you really want to be set free? Then let go of control, focus on the leading of God in the area of eating, and enjoy a thin body and normal eating habits.

What You Can Do Today

- Go where God is leading you in Scripture.

- *Never be afraid to question anything that seems contrary to God's design.* Do you feel confused by all the "lose-weight-quick" fads, harsh diets, or pills on the market? Remember that there is nothing wrong with debate. In fact, questioning an issue will get you deeper into God's Word and help you find a deeper understanding. Search God's Word for *His* truth before accepting the "truth" of whatever fad is popular at the time.

- *Examine man-made rules.* The next time you hear a food rule, do not hesitate to question it. Compare it to God's Word and the rules He gives us to live by. When you have faith in the way He created your body to work, you won't be as quick to believe the man-made rules.

- *Share God's awesome plan for eating.* The next time you hear a close friend or family member considering a desperate measure to lose weight, such as using dangerous diet pills or undergoing risky surgery that alters God's system of digestion, take a moment to talk with him about God's plan for eating. Share with him about the hunger mechanism and the way God programmed the body to know when, what, and how much to eat, just as He programmed it to know when, what, and how much to breathe. Let him know there is a truthful alternative to the desperate measures.

- *Make a commitment to stop dieting.* Stop doing anything that makes you talk about, focus on, or lust after food ever again.

_____

_____

_____

_____

How to Eat Steak, a Baked Potato, and Dessert

My friends and I love to celebrate a special occasion with a wonderful steak dinner. I might skip lunch to make sure that I am really, *really* hungry! When the meal arrives at the table, I eat the best morsels while they are hot, remembering to save room for my favorite dessert. Plenty of real butter and sour cream for my baked potato assures that I can create the perfect combination. First, I sprinkle salt and pepper on the potato. I love salt! Next, I add the butter, and then I top it off with a lot of sour cream—and I mean a lot! I then move on to the medium-rare filet mignon. I cut until I reach the center, which has the juiciest pieces. As soon as I select the "prime cut," I add a small amount of salt. The filet that is cooked right will just melt in your mouth. After alternating several bites of baked potato, filet, and salad with blue cheese dressing, I am comfortably satisfied. Since I have eaten only the *best* bites, my plate looks like something I dissected in a lab class because all the dry, unseasoned, or just short of perfect pieces have been left behind! As I enjoy the company of my friends, I push my plate aside with the half-eaten baked potato and filet. I ask for a carryout and take it home for a nice meal the next day. I occasionally pass on dessert, but not this night! A special occasion calls for the ultimate brownie topped with hot caramel, chocolate fudge, whipped cream, nuts— and several spoons for sharing! Again, I search for the perfect bite before the towering dessert begins to melt. A few sips of coffee, a lot of laughter, and a couple of bites from the brownie add the perfect ending to a memorable evening among friends. I am indeed comfortably satisfied. I praise God for the friends more than I do for the food, but both are great, and He is awesome!

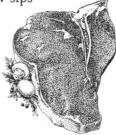

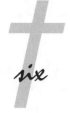

six

SECRET OF THE PRISON

To open eyes that are blind,
to free captives from prison
and to release from the dungeon those who sit in darkness.
—Isaiah 42:7

I am so excited that you have been given a vision of more freedom in Christ and have decided to go on this journey with us—from the prison of things on this earth into a freedom where nothing in this world has a hold on your heart, mind, or soul. There are many lies in the prison of overweight, and we are going on a journey through the Word of God so you will discover the true secret of this dungeon. God is guiding you into a closer walk with Him. I challenge you to continue the journey because there is more to be had. God is waking up His people to show us that He loves us and expects more love from each of us. In many ways, I believe that God is judging His people right *now,* so it is time to examine your freedom in Christ or your slavery to the world.

After you have been overweight for a long time, you start to read and believe the graffiti lies that have been written by prisoners who are enslaved for life. They have no plans to get out, so they don't want *you* free, either. Why not listen to someone who is free? I have

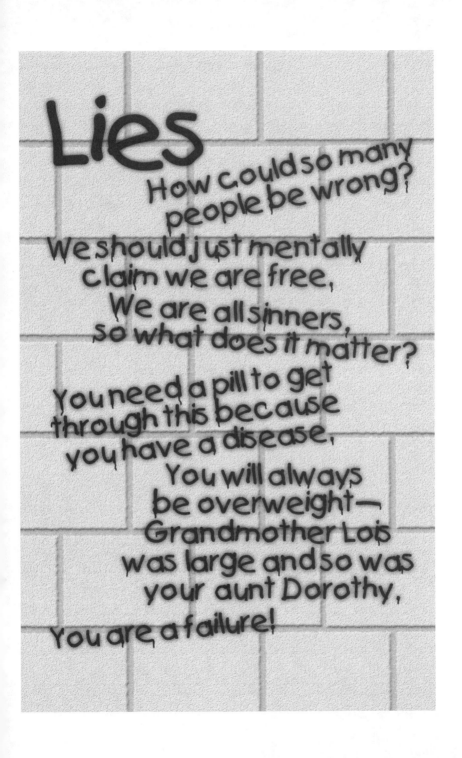

Lies

How could so many
people be wrong?

We should just mentally
claim we are free,
We are all sinners,
so what does it matter?

You need a pill to get
through this because
you have a disease,
You will always
be overweight—
Grandmother Lois
was large and so was
your aunt Dorothy,

You are a failure!

not been overweight for approximately twenty years. I am free from the pull of extra food, diets, diet pills, "have-to" exercise programs, suction-assisted lipectomies, meal exchanges, and low-fat foods. I am free to eat blue cheese dressing, cheesecake, real bacon, hamburgers and French fries, and more. There are no restricted foods unless you have a special medical condition or allergy. I have worn the same skirts for twenty years. I am free from having to focus on foods or my body or weight. I have remained the same size simply because of a choice of what I worship or adore. I love the Creator and His will (moderation) more than the created (the food).

Let's review some of the truths that Jesus said will set us free. In John 8, Jesus said, "If you hold to my teaching, you are really my disciples. [Some people are really not His disciples.] *Then* you will know the truth, and the truth *will set you free....* I tell you the truth, everyone who sins is a slave to sin. Now a slave has no permanent place in the family, but a son belongs to it forever. So if the Son sets you free, you will be free indeed" (vv. 31b–32, 34–36, italics added). If you are still struggling with your weight or any sin, notice the progression Jesus teaches: (1) *"If* you hold to my teaching..." (2) *"then* you will know the truth" (not before)... and (3) *then* "the truth will set you free."

If you are struggling, then this book will help you examine Jesus' teachings vs. Satan's counterfeit church teachings, and it will help you apply those of Jesus. You will then *know—know* the truth—and the truth will set you free!

I believe the truth is that we all have been enslaved to something on this earth. We all have been in Egypt and enslaved as the children of God were, but God promised in Genesis that He would surely bring us out. Notice that the only ones who followed God out of Egypt were the Israelites who had been enslaved. Everyone else remained in Egypt and even did his best to keep the children of God from leaving. Those who remained thought that slavery to this world was great—*after all,* they thought, *everyone else is enslaved.* If you are in slavery to food, you may think dieting is great—after all, everyone else is on the same kind of diet. To pull away from what everyone else is doing seems scary, but it will set you free!

GRAFFITI LIE #1:
How Could So Many People Be Wrong?

This brings up the first graffiti lie written on the prison cell: How could so many people be wrong? It's the volume lie—the highway lie. But you must combat the highway lie with the truth of Jesus. Stay in the Word from God—the One who gets it all! Jesus said, "Enter through the narrow gate. For wide is the gate and broad is the road that leads to destruction, and many enter through it. But small is the gate and narrow the road that leads to life, and only a few find it" (Matt. 7:13–14). Jesus Himself walked a lonely path if you count numbers—but a full path if you consider that God was by His side. Stop feeling lonely, and begin to feel popular and blessed from a heavenly standard.

How could so many people be wrong? It's the volume lie—the highway lie.

There will always be two voices, so you *must know:* (1) there are two forces—good and evil, and (2) you must search for the truth. Jesus said again and again, "I tell you *the* truth." Stay in the Word, and don't run away from hard teachings because they will unlock your *heart.*

If preachers or Christian authors are telling you that certain foods are bad for you, quote them the truth. Jesus said, "'For it doesn't go into his heart but into his stomach, and then out of his body.' (In saying this, Jesus declared all foods 'clean.')" (Mark 7:19). The Apostle Paul wrote,

The Spirit clearly says that in later times some will abandon the faith and follow deceiving spirits and things taught by demons. Such

teachings come through hypocritical liars, whose consciences have been seared as with a hot iron. They forbid people to marry and order them to abstain from certain foods, which God created to be received with thanksgiving by those who believe and who know the truth. For everything God created is good, and nothing is to be rejected if it is received with thanksgiving. (1 Tim. 4:1–4)

That is God's *truth.* If the food were evil, then it would take the responsibility away from the heart of mankind—and this is the masterpiece lie of Satan that keeps you behind prison walls. So please realize: *it is not the food's fault!*

"Everyone else is dieting and exercising to lose weight. Maybe I am wrong!?" No—but it *will* often seem as if you are against the world. But you can show the world the fruit that comes from concentrating on making the heart pure. That fruit is *weight loss,* which comes from eating only what the body truly calls for, not what your hands or mouth wants.

GRAFFITI LIE #2:
We Should Just Mentally Claim We Are Free.

A part of God's plan is for us to realize the vulnerable state of our hearts and how easy it is for us to get entangled in this world—and how *right* it is to fight to choose daily the way that we should go. We don't just claim our freedom—we must obey God and fight daily battles.

I am simply a servant of yours. I am not above you, for God has sent me to work for you, to think about your needs, and to concentrate on how I can motivate you to seek, love, and obey Him more. Nothing makes me happy but to get up every day and say, "Thank You for letting me live—it didn't have to be me. Now, what do You want me to do today?" Just as the Bible states in John 4:34, "'My food,' said Jesus, 'is to do the will of him who sent me and to finish his work,'" I can't wait to totally translate to you this rock-solid foundational attitude that keeps me happy, peaceful, *and* full of purpose. But you must get prepared for battle, for you are a soldier of Christ. Welcome to the army of the kingdom of God!

The Bible talks a lot about "high places" or strongholds—things we cling to in order to cope with this ever-changing orbiting world where the winds change *daily!* "High places" are mentioned more than sixty times in the Bible. Remember, the children of Israel held on to Egypt and they could not get out on their own, but God rescued them, taking them to the desert of testing and finally to the Promised Land. In the Promised Land, there is less competition for your heart because your heart has chosen to worship and adore only God, and it no longer desires your past strongholds. The Promised Land is where the heart has transferred its passion. It craves only approval and love from the Father and Jesus Christ, His Son. The children of Israel, once in the Promised Land, would take over territory for the kingdom of God (Deut. 7:22–24). God deserves to be the Ruler of *all*—not just a few. You must stay awake in the Promised Land. Paul described the whole lifelong journey as a *race*—running for the prize (1 Cor. 9:24).

GRAFFITI LIE #3:
We Are All Sinners, So What Does It Matter?

As you've learned by now, Weigh Down† is simply mere Christianity, and the seminars are simply gatherings of the sheep or lambs of God. Many of the counterfeit teachings that are out today are so discouraging and rob you of your freedom. They leave you feeling as if you will *never* be free from overindulging your particular bad habit. After all, the false teachings say, we are all sinners and we will all continue in sin that grace may abound (Rom. 6:1, 5; 1 Cor. 15:10; 2 Cor. 9:8).

Yes, it is true that we all have sinned. I have sinned. We all have sinned and hurt the heart of the Father. But Jesus came to set you free so that you might glorify a powerful God who brings life to dry bones (Ezek. 37). We are called to repent and be a royal and holy priesthood of believers and a pure bride for Christ. First Peter 4:1–2 tells us, "Therefore, since Christ suffered in his body, arm yourselves also with the same attitude, because he who has suffered in his body is done with sin. As a result, he does not live the rest of his earthly life for evil human desires, but rather for the will of God."

I have witnessed thousands of people embrace this cross through Weigh Down† and walk free from sexual lust, extra food, overdrinking, excessive TV, anger, or the pursuit of money. I have witnessed people walk away from cigarettes, being a control-freak, homosexuality, anorexia, and bulimia. They have walked free from workaholism, laziness, gambling, depression, materialism, hate, jealousy, self-pity, phobias, and panic attacks. I have seen them set free from selfish ambition, boasting, selfishness, slander, and pride. Individuals walking free—even after being in prison for fifty years. Walking free—*never* to return to their old habits. This is living proof that an even stronger magnetic pull is out there somewhere!

God *is* real. There are so many people walking free in Weigh Down† classes after having been in prison on many a church pew because they had bought the sweet-sounding "tickle-your-ear" lie that we are all just a building full of "continue in sin" sinners. Why? Because I warn them that they are set-free saints whose *past* sins and *stumbling* sins are washed and covered by the blood of Jesus. We are not to *continue* in sin that grace may abound. Romans 6:1b–2a states clearly, "Shall we go on sinning so that grace may increase? *By no means!*" (italics added).

> I have witnessed thousands of people embrace this cross through Weigh Down† and walk free from sexual lust, extra food, overdrinking, excessive TV, anger, or the pursuit of money.

I am not special—I am no different from anyone else. If I seem to be free to love God, it is only due to the fact that when I'm tempted, I get down on my knees, flat on my face before God and in His Word, and surrender. Then I surrender a little more. Then I surrender it all—until the Lord shows me the next level of death. But do I *look* dead? No! *Life* comes from dying to your own will and replacing it with God's will—not your spouse's or boss's or kids' wishes, but *God's will.*

As time has gone by it has become easier to make good choices because I increasingly see the results or consequences—both negative and positive—that have affected my entire life and the lives of those around me when I obey or disobey the Father. Each of us has been given a heart that is capable of making a choice in its devotion. We will have either a Cain attitude or an Abel attitude. Cain wanted God to accept whatever sacrifice he chose to give, while Abel sacrificed the very finest he had to offer—the best of the best (Gen. 4:3–5). We have the ability to choose which attitude we will have.

We are told to "master sin" by Genesis 4, and we are told to repent or else in Revelation. We are told to "walk in the light." First John 1:6–7 states, "If we claim to have fellowship with him yet walk in the darkness, we lie and do not live by the truth. But if we *walk in the light,* as he is in the light, we have fellowship with one another, and the blood of Jesus, his Son, purifies us from all sin" (italics added). Walking implies an action that we all can learn to do. This passage implies choice—do not walk in the darkness. When you walk in the light of Jesus Christ, you can compare yourself to His attitudes, and this plumb line shows your imperfections. The passage continues, "If we confess our sins, he is faithful and just and will forgive us our sins and purify us" (1 John 1:9). But John went on to write,

My dear children, I write this to you so that you will not sin. . . . Dear children, do not let anyone lead you astray. He who does what is right is righteous, just as he is righteous. He who does what is sinful is of

the devil, because the devil has been sinning from the beginning. The reason the Son of God appeared was to destroy the devil's work. No one who is born of God will continue to sin, because God's seed remains in him; he cannot go on sinning, because he has been born of God. This is how we know who the children of God are and who the children of the devil are: Anyone who does not do what is right is not a child of God; nor is anyone who does not love his brother. (1 John 2:1; 3:7–10)

Second Peter tells us we have been given *everything* we need for life and godliness (2 Peter 1:3).

GRAFFITI LIE #4:
You Need a Pill to Get Through This Because You Have a Disease.

The Bible does not say you need Jesus Christ *and* a pill to be set free. Remember, pills, regimented exercise, dieting, and self-focused therapy have never helped anyone die to self and desire less food. Unfortunately, most health professionals and self-help groups still teach that you have a disease and that the rest of your life will be affected by the disease. "Once an alcoholic, always an alcoholic." "Once a bulimic, always a bulimic." Once "patients" are diagnosed with panic attacks, depression, or bulimia, the disease is considered essentially chronic. They are told that obesity is inherited, genetic, congenital, and it is their mothers' fault, and that they have to count fat grams and deny themselves fat and sweets for the rest of their lives. How enslaving!

By the 1980s, I grew encouraged. It seemed that psychological organizations were getting closer to the answer because they started addressing behavior modification. They said that changing your behavior is the answer, but they never gave any successful advice on how to make the change permanent because they never included the

God of our behavior—in whose likeness we were created. This god-less behavior modification left clients feeling like failures because they could not just up and stop smoking, overeating, gambling, having panic attacks, or having affairs. I personally experienced failure at weight loss, and I repeatedly attempted to change my behavior by using fat grams, low-carbohydrate diets, exchange lists, and increased exercise. I did what they told me and parked my car in the most faraway parking place, among many other things.

The next step—of course, in this country—is to treat the condition with pills, patches, formulas, or surgery because you must have an irregular chemical imbalance or unfortunate genetic makeup that excuses your inability to cope or overcome your phobias and unwanted behaviors.

By the grace of God, I found out that changing my behavior was going to require a power much stronger than the simple determination of mankind and a few suggestions from a white coat. Never did I find even one piece of medical literature that was humble enough—much less wise enough—to admit that this power comes only from God Almighty. God had been left out of the books, or God or Jesus was mixed in with a pill or exchange groups or "have-to" lifetime therapy groups. "Jesus/God plus _____ (fill in the blank) = freedom."

It really took many years for me to understand how to express the connection that God Almighty has to unlocking the strongholds. But eventually, God moved me to write, speak, and offer help using His truths. I sat in a counseling room and told people if they wanted to be set free from overweight, they should eat food only when they were physiologically hungry. Then I told them that when they still had the desire to overeat at ten o'clock at night when no one was looking, they

It really took many years for me to understand how to express the connection that God Almighty does have to unlocking the strongholds.

When my wife asked me to attend a Weigh Down[†] class with her, I was working out more aggressively than I had in years, punishing my body with low-fat and no-satisfaction dieting, and getting nowhere. I knew I could no longer control my problem and felt hopeless. My background as a physical therapist had taught me about caloric needs, body types, and metabolism, but never why overweight people like myself were so tormented over food. Through this wonderful program, God has truly changed our lives and given us a peace about food. Praise God!

Mark & Lisa Ware—Brandon, MS
Mark lost 60 lbs.—Lisa lost 38 lbs.

I resisted starting the program, rationalizing that I would not be successful because my weight problem was hereditary. I could not exercise due to left-side paralysis from recurrent strokes, and it really didn't matter how large I was in a wheelchair. But through Weigh Down[†], God freed me of 110 pounds, and it has remained off for 2 years.

June Vaughn—Bruce, MS
Lost 110 lbs., from size 24 to size 8
and has kept it off 2 years

Whenever I would say anything about my weight, people would say, "It's not your fault. You just can't exercise." But, praise the Lord, through Weigh Down[†] I have gone from a size 22 to a size 5 with no exercise!

Tammie Walker—Anaheim, CA
Lost about 100 lbs.,
from size 22 to size 5
and has kept it off 2 years

should chew on *this*—and I would hand them a Bible. Many would lose weight permanently. I encouraged them to apply this concept to any stronghold. Critics who were unaware of the foundation of what I taught would continually say, "What does God have to do with weight loss or smoking?" or "They will never make it if they let people eat red meat and fat, and everyone *knows* you have to exercise to stay skinny." Lies, lies, lies.

Lies are written all over the prison walls. Anyone saying these things is still a prisoner. Anyone still in prison has not found God's Escape Route—*Jesus plus* nothing, *thank you!*

Well, all strongholds are a matter of the heart. And God is the Maker of the heart. He is the major heart Surgeon—and He is the Pursuer of our hearts. This behavior change belongs in the hands of God and in His Word.

When you search for solutions in the Word of God, you learn that there is a big tug-of-war for our devotion, and many things can steal our hearts. But there is only one place where our hearts belong, and that is in a submissive, slavelike state before Jesus Christ. Please know that I am a happy slave to God and righteousness! Romans 6:16 teaches us, "Don't you know that when you offer yourselves to someone to obey him as slaves, you are slaves to the one whom you obey—whether you are slaves to sin, which leads to death, or to obedience, which leads to righteousness?" We are all made to be slaves to something, and I can overwhelmingly endorse *this* Slave Master!

We can give our hearts to man and try to get the praise and approval of man. We can depend on doctors, therapists, pills, diets, exercise, throwing up food, laxatives, celery, and home exercise machines. We can escape and get busy with sports, TV, our children, our work, or the pursuit of money. We can even escape with the work at the church building. But we somehow resist Jesus because He walked straight toward a death sentence—but He is now on the right-hand side of God. We have sneaky, wriggly, resistant hearts, and it is time for America (and especially God's church) to stop fearing the cross. Stop wearing it on your neck and wrist if you do not really mean it.

Once you see this clearly, you will be able to make moves and choices that you have never, ever been able to do—not even under intense medical therapy and drugs (especially under the therapy of drugs!). And once you begin to make these choices, you will see that nothing is impossible and there is nothing to fear when your focus is only on God Almighty.

A doctor here in Nashville was doing some routine surgery on a patient's shoulder when suddenly and totally unexpectedly, the patient's heart stopped beating. The doctor began manually pumping the heart, giving artificial respiration, and administering medications. He ordered the heart defibrillator, an electric shock treatment, for the patient sixteen times—a number that is dangerously over the normal number administered. After sixty minutes of trying, the cardiologist assisting with the effort suggested that the frantic doctor give up, but he kept working. At an hour and fifteen minutes, the cardiologist again said that enough had been done, and again, the doctor continued to force air into the lungs and massage the heart. The clock kept ticking. At an hour and a half, the cardiologist spoke a third time about the futility of continuing, and with complete exhaustion, the doctor finally agreed, gave up, and took his hands off the patient. He had done all he could do—far beyond the call of duty. They all reluctantly stepped back from the table and began putting equipment away.

Suddenly, they heard a sound. *What is this? Could it be the heart monitor?* Yes, the patient's heart was beating and he was breathing! Within minutes, the patient had regained consciousness and could hear the doctor speaking. Extensive testing revealed that this man— who had been clinically dead and had undergone ninety minutes of incomplete oxygen to his brain—had suffered no memory loss and no physical or mental problems at all! He didn't even show signs of heart damage or bruising that is common with lengthy CPR and multiple electric shocks. The doctor gave all credit to God and even stated that he believed the ninety minutes of futile effort were part of God's plan. He later told a local newspaper, "It was as if God was saying, 'Step back. *I* am the Great Physician. Let me show you what real healing power is.'"[1]

This story was picked up by national media and was a great way to put God on the front page. God plus nothing. When we do not call upon the Creator, our work is like the work of a two-year-old helping clean the house. We mess up more quickly than we can possibly help. But when we acknowledge God, we can do miraculous things!

America needs faith and humility to get out of this prison of obesity. It is sad that some practitioners fail to see that God is not going to bless their hands as long as they continue to leave Him out. Again, not to belabor the point, there are other clinics that do include God with a "seek ye fifth" or "seek ye sixth" treatment protocol instead of *"seek ye first* the kingdom of God and His righteousness," as the Bible teaches us. In other words, they depend mainly on the man-made treatments, and God is simply added to the list. This can be spiritually deflating to a person who feels as if he has used a Christ-centered approach, but yet he is no better for it. God is insisting that godless, man-made rules for a disciplined life will not work. Look at Colossians 2:22–23:

> *These [rules] are all destined to perish with use, because they are based on human commands and teachings. Such regulations indeed have an appearance of wisdom, with their self-imposed worship, their false humility and their harsh treatment of the body, but they lack any value in restraining sensual indulgence.*

When spiritual issues and sensual indulgence are not tackled or addressed and redirected using the good news of Jesus Christ, then

America needs faith and humility to get out of this prison of obesity.

all we have are man-made rules. You will know that you are apply-ing man-made solutions if they do not help redirect the heart of man. Man-made rules can turn your world into a monastery, and yet a monastery cannot keep your behavior pure. A heart could be pure in a monastery, or it could be pure out in the world. On the other hand, a heart can entertain evil, greedy thoughts inside a monastery, or a heart could entertain lust when it is in worldly places. The key is a pure, clean heart. First Peter 1:22a states, "You have purified your-selves by *obeying the truth.*"

Speaking of labeling our actions a "disease"—the term *anorexia nervosa* wasn't even a medical term before 1870. But when practi-tioners in the 1980s or 1990s come up with a disease-sounding label, such as *anorexia nervosa* or *alcoholism* or *bulimia* or *agoraphobia* or *compulsive anything,* they are trying to take a spiritual problem and label it as a disease—and if it is a disease, then it most often follows that it is out of our control. Now why would a doctor want to label so many spiritual problems as a "disease"? Because it takes it out of the hands of God and puts it in the hospitals and counseling centers. You become dependent on those people, pills, and procedures. You could agree that the love of money is the root of *many* evils.

Present professional industries all too often misdirect the broken-hearted by teaching them that they have a special and rare condition or a unique dysfunctional family problem. Since it is now a disease, then the people or families do not battle these problems in an effec-tive way. The professionals make them feel as if they need special medical treatment, counsel, or pills for their spiritual problems. Wrong, wrong, wrong. "Rare" is finding someone with a pure single-minded heart for Jesus Christ and God Almighty—someone who knows already to feed off the pastures of Jehovah only, and not something on this earth (Jer. 50:5–6). In fact, it just so happens that every human at one point or another in life lusts after or adores something on this earth more than God. That is the definition of *sin.* We are free to enjoy all of God's earth—just not to worship it.

GRAFFITI LIE #5:
You Will Always Be Overweight. Grandmother Lois Was Large, and so Was Your Aunt Dorothy.

The only person who never lost His focus, who never had any ambition but to make God known and admired, and whose full feeling was found in doing the will of the Father was Jesus Christ. Do not feel alone—you are not different. This is a fallen world. But we have been called to rise above the world—to come out of the world, to be holy as God is holy, to purify ourselves, and to be *like* Christ. We have been given a heart that can make a choice—it is called responsibility—and the spirit of Christ in our hearts has that resurrection power. *Responsibility* means we have the *ability* to make a *response.* Don't listen to the lies of Satan that say, "Grandmother Lois was large, and so was your aunt Dorothy." It is this prison lie that gives Americans a big invitation to binge. Even godless countries do not have this attitude, and Americans are known for their self-indulgence (the opposite of being Christlike). Satan loves to wreak havoc in a country that claims "In God We Trust" on every dollar bill.

Again, the basis of any stronghold is a heart that is misplaced. It loves the gambling or the alcohol, or it feels alive or fulfilled with sexual lust or the pursuit of money or power, or it feels as if it is happier with the drugs or cigarettes or extra food. Misplaced hearts are all alike, and they can all be set free through Christ.

I am here today to tell you it is not that complicated or difficult. The road to freedom is not expensive and does not require unusual ongoing therapy. You just have to want out of your present situation, and you have to look for and seek God. That is it. You can do this. You just have to want out and turn to God for help and cry out to Him—not for just one day, but a lifelong, eternity-long attitude of dependence.

GRAFFITI LIE #6:
You Are a Failure Because You Have Not Lost Weight.

I have good news. Even though you have tried many times to quit your bad habit, you are not a failure. You are the exact opposite—you are a prize to be won, and there are two forces fighting over you: the forces of the evil world and the forces of heaven above. Both the evil force and the good force want your heart and soul. Now, just why would both forces want you so badly if you are a "nothing" or a "failure"? Indeed, you are very valuable—so valuable that much has gone into the planning and executing of even getting your heart to beat, so valuable that God has invested in an attentive heavenly staff to help you along, grow you, test you, and keep you from the evil forces (Job 7:17–19).

Both the evil force and the good force want your heart and soul. Now, just why would both forces want you so badly if you are a "nothing" or a "failure"?

Yes, you have tried to quit smoking, cussing, stealing, lying, being lazy, watching too much TV, lusting, hating, or being negative or depressed, but you have just not been able to overcome. No, you are not really happy, and many a day you would like to end your life or you wish that God would save you the trouble and do it for you. Self-mutilation to make you "feel better" is whispered in the ear by Satan. But just because you are not happy, that does not mean that you are not valuable. Remember, you are a prize to be won. This lack of happiness you are feeling comes from misdirected dedication and effort in life. It comes from not directing all your energy toward a give-and-take relationship with God. The unhappiness comes from not taking the time to comprehend how wonderful it is to be in good with the only Person we should be in good with—and that is the invisible God of the universe.

You will experience inexpressible joy and peace when you finally understand that you have an opportunity to be promoted to the largest corporation of the universe, that you get to join the most prestigious army of the world, that you get to be married (see marriage symbolism in 2 Cor. 11:2; Rev. 19:7; 21:2) to the best-looking and most-loving and richest Husband of all times, or that you get to be best friends with the most coordinated top Athlete of every sport: baseball, football, wrestling, soccer, basketball, swimming, gymnastics, and track. You have the opportunity to be connected to the richest Banker there ever was or ever will be, and you are able to get to know and use the healing hand of the number one intellectual Genius and medical Physician of all times.

In addition, you can actually approach the presence of this most powerful Being. He is the Master of the wind, the land, and the seas, and He is the Master of all living creatures. As children, we were enchanted when Tarzan could command the obedience of the animals in the jungle, but God's power can command man and beast and all the elements of the universe to do His will. This kind of power can raise dead people and make their hearts beat again and can create new people. It can make the earth split apart and quake, and it can hold the vast earth in orbit in space. It is power that can even reach down and teach a tiny colony of ants (who have a microchip for a brain) to organize and prepare for upcoming winter weather.

With just a moment to contemplate this enchanting Hero, you can be moved to worship, and when you are moved to worship God, you will no longer worship your stronghold, and you find the power to walk free. As time goes on, you realize that He knows the exact number of hairs on your head. You are drawn in to love Him, for you finally realize there is no person, place, or thing that can love you the way He can. His demands are highly rewarded.

This journey gives you a chance to find Him, and the Bible says that "the LORD searches every heart and understands every motive behind

If you seek him, he will be found by you, but if you forsake him, he will reject you forever.

(1 Chron. 28:9b)

the thoughts. If you seek him, he will be found by you, but if you forsake him, he will reject you forever" (1 Chron. 28:9b). So, if you will seek Him with all of your heart, you will find Him. It makes me lose my breath to think that I am touching the edges of the garment of finding Him. It makes me lose my breath to think about losing His favor or being rejected by Him. I want to know the meaning of *seeking,* and I want to know the meaning of *forsaking.*

SO WHAT DO WE DO?

What is the appropriate response toward this powerful Being? First, we need to stop trying to blame the world around us and make the environment change. Satan's biggest legalistic attack on the church is that the things around us are evil. Satan even wants us to believe that certain foods are evil. If we don't know good from evil, we can never know what to do. Micah 3 shows us that God became angry with leaders who did not know good from evil:

> Listen, you leaders of Jacob,
>> you rulers of the house of Israel.
> Should you not know justice,
>> you who hate good and love evil? (Mic. 3:1–2a)

It is basic theology to know what is clean and unclean—what God's will is. In other words, removing all the alcohol, fat grams, and tempting chocolate from the house is not really the answer. Sending the family to counseling to make them change and accept your deviant behavior is not the answer. Making the environment clean up or the people around you change will never change your own heart.

Jesus taught that it was not the environment that needed to change, but the heart of man. Really meditate on this foundational Weigh Down^t passage in Mark 7:

> *Again Jesus called the crowd to him and said, "Listen to me, everyone, and understand this. Nothing outside a man can make him 'unclean' by going into him. Rather, it is what comes out of a man that makes him 'unclean.'" After he had left the crowd and entered the house, his disciples asked him about this parable. "Are you so dull?" he asked. "Don't you see that nothing that enters a man from the outside can make him 'unclean'? For it doesn't go into his heart but into his stomach, and then out of his body." (In saying this, Jesus declared all foods "clean.") He went on: "What comes out of a man is what makes him 'unclean.' For from within, out of men's hearts, come evil thoughts, sexual immorality, theft, murder, adultery, greed, malice, deceit, lewdness, envy, slander, arrogance and folly. All these evils come from inside and make a man 'unclean.'" (vv. 14–23)*

I spent so much of my life thinking that alcohol was unclean that I was scared to even touch a bottle. I thought that fat or red meat was evil. It never dawned on me to be afraid of the evil in my own heart. My own lusts separated me from getting the Father's love and answered prayers, yet no one preached this truth. Many teachers today spend their time on legalistic man-made rules for the church. There has been so much wasted guilt on things that God would love for us to enjoy, yet no guilt at all over the things we do that make God mad or angry. The body of Christ as a whole in the 30,000 churches where Weigh Down^t has been taught was shocked to hear that God loves brownies! The false rumors of God keep people distant from Him. Who wants to get to know a God who hates chocolate brownies?!

Making the environment clean up or the people around you change will never change your own heart.

We have become experts at changing the content of food by pulling out the fat and throwing in some tasteless fiber, pulling the alcohol out of beer, trying to clean up the schools, the government, or the music industry, and so on and so forth. However, we are completely at a loss when it comes to changing our own hearts so that we no longer have a stronghold. Genesis 4:6–7 tells us: "Then the LORD said to Cain, 'Why are you angry? Why is your face downcast? If you do what is right, will you not be accepted? But if you do not do what is right, sin is crouching at your door; it desires to have you, but you must master it.'"

We have spent all of our energy on cleaning up the wrong things. Jesus said not to take the splinter out of someone else's eye when we have a log in our own. We must first take the log out of our own eye; then we can see clearly to remove the speck out of someone else's eye. We are scared of the things on this earth, but what *should* scare us are the unclean things that God reveals about our own hearts. The heart is what is greedy. The alcohol is not evil—God created it. The drug is not evil. The food is not evil. Sex is not evil. Tobacco is not evil. It is the *worship* of it that is evil. Worship is focus and adoration. We worship these things. It is what you are drooling over in your heart that should bring you to your knees because you can get the alcohol out of the house or the fat grams out of the house, but you cannot run from your own heart and mind. And your heart and mind face the Judgment Day. You must change and pray—pray hard—for a cleansing from the Father through Jesus Christ.

On behalf of people living in the last few decades, let's concede that we have never been told that we have a heart problem. I have a master's degree in foods and nutrition, and yet we *never* studied the greed in the heart of mankind. We only dissected the content of the foods and labeled each ingredient as clean or unclean. Again, my experience has been that most of the churches have bought into the man-made "clean" and "unclean" rules. Everyone confidently and self-righteously preached that broccoli was righteous, and that brownies and ice cream were sinful. But now we know the truth. The food is clean—God just wants our hearts to be clean.

HOW TO START LOSING WEIGHT AGAIN

Remember to review the basics of the Weigh Down Workshop[†] program in Appendix A and Appendix B of this book. But know that you can get started right now. An important part of the process of repentance includes the recognition that our relationship with God is wounded if our hearts are unclean—in other words, if our hearts secretly long for or lust for something else on this earth—for more, that is, than what the Father has allotted. If we are plotting for, longing for, or wanting something on this earth, then we cannot be plotting for, longing for, or wanting *God* with all of our hearts. We can have only one master and love of our lives. All other false gods or idols in our lives should pale next to the true, awesome, and coordinated God of the universe. So in other words, the first major step is to recognize that you have been trying to clean up everything else—all in the name of God, of course—and you had no idea that cleaning up your own heart is the major job description God has given you.

The second step is to realize that if even a piece of your heart is not right, it is hurting God's heart, and it prevents a wholehearted relationship with God. Anytime someone or something besides God has hold of your heart, it is sin. Instead of making a list of specific things, learn that you can feel it in your heart. If you are attached to any person, anything, or any behavior that you cannot seem to stop, that is a heart attachment—a stronghold—and you need to let go and cling to God or just wait on God. Jonah 2:8 states that "those who cling to worthless idols forfeit the grace that could be theirs."

The third major step is to turn your mind and heart and soul to God—turn to God any way you know how. You need to direct your sensitivity toward God and away from the stronghold. Exodus 20 gives God's perspective on this matter:

I am the LORD your God, who brought you out of Egypt, out of the
land of slavery. You shall have no other gods before me. You shall not
make for yourself an idol in the form of anything in heaven above or
on the earth beneath or in the waters below. You shall not bow down
to them or worship them; for I, the LORD your God, am a jealous God,
punishing the children for the sin of the fathers to the third and fourth
generation of those who hate me, but showing love to a thousand gen-
erations of those who love me and keep my commandments. (vv. 2–6)

You were born to worship and you do worship. What is on your
mind all the time is your idol; it is what you adore. But you need to
adore Jesus Christ. So we've established that you will give your heart,
soul, mind, and strength to *something*—and that is worship. In fact,
you could even call it addiction. But, again, you were born to do this,
so, actually, being addicted is normal. And I am not asking you not
to be addicted. I am asking you to be addicted to something that can
love you back, and there is only One who can do that—our heavenly
Father through Jesus Christ, His Son.

We have learned something. Hurting God's heart and causing Him
to be jealous are sin. Now we can look for what the Bible has to say
about sin or idolatry, something we had no idea we were committing. The first place to stop is the sixth chapter of Romans. It says,
"What shall we say, then? Shall we go on sinning so that grace may
increase? By no means!" (Rom. 6:1–2a). The Bible says *by no means.*
They were discussing the very thing we are discussing two thousand
years later! The question is still, "What does God expect from us?"
Let's continue reading:

We died to sin; how can we live in it any longer? Or don't you know
that all of us who were baptized into Christ Jesus were baptized into
his death? We were therefore buried with him through baptism into
death in order that, just as Christ was raised from the dead through
the glory of the Father, we too may live a new life. If we have been

united with him like this in his death, we will certainly also be united with him in his resurrection. For we know that our old self was crucified with him so that the body of sin might be done away with, that we should no longer be slaves to sin—because anyone who has died has been freed from sin. (Rom. 6:2b–7)

So when we come to the Father through Jesus Christ, we die to our old lovers and say "yes" to our new love, God Almighty. We are free from sin—in other words, free to love God.

We are under grace, the Apostle Paul said, but he then continued, "What then? Shall we sin because we are not under law but under grace? By no means!" The text here includes one of the rare exclamation marks. "By no means!" Paul went on to say,

Don't you know that when you offer yourselves to someone to obey him as slaves, you are slaves to the one whom you obey—whether you are slaves to sin, which leads to death, or to obedience, which leads to righteousness? . . . You have been set free from sin and have become slaves to righteousness. . . . Just as you used to offer the parts of your body in slavery to impurity and to ever-increasing wickedness, so now offer them in slavery to righteousness leading to holiness. When you were slaves to sin, you were free from the control of righteousness. What benefit did you reap at that time from the things you are now ashamed of? Those things result in death! But now that you have been set free from sin and have become slaves to God, the benefit you reap leads to holiness, and the result is eternal life. (Rom. 6:15–16, 18, 19b–22)

Being addicted is normal. I am not asking you not to be addicted. I am asking you to be addicted to something that can love you back.

And look at this passage from Ephesians 4:

So I tell you this, and insist on it in the Lord, that you must no longer live as the Gentiles do, in the futility of their thinking. They are darkened in their understanding and separated from the life of God because of the ignorance that is in them due to the hardening of their hearts. Having lost all sensitivity, they have given themselves over to sensuality so as to indulge in every kind of impurity, with a continual lust for more. You, however, did not come to know Christ that way. Surely you heard of him and were taught in him in accordance with the truth that is in Jesus. You were taught, with regard to your former way of life, to put off your old self, which is being corrupted by its deceitful desires; to be made new in the attitude of your minds; and to put on the new self, created to be like God in true righteousness and holiness. (vv. 17–24)

Notice from this passage that continuing in sin separates you from God. We were never expected to continue in sin. When I first started writing and speaking, I would cry out to God that these passages seemed stronger than what I heard being preached. I did not want to be the bearer of bad news or strict news. But then I would open to a passage that was even clearer and stricter than the first, such as this one from 1 John 3:6: "No one who lives in him keeps on sinning. No one who continues to sin has either seen him or known him."

And in the book of Titus, it says:

For the grace of God that brings salvation has appeared to all men. It teaches us to say "No" to ungodliness and worldly passions, and to live self-controlled, upright and godly lives in this present age, while we wait for the blessed hope—the glorious appearing of our great God and Savior, Jesus Christ, who gave himself for us to redeem us from all wickedness and to purify for himself a people that are his very own, eager to do what is good. (Titus 2:11–14)

So all along, the grace of God was to teach us to say "No," and to repent and turn, and to do what is good.

I am not sure where we got this idea that we can come to the Lord without repentance. But perhaps the confusion over the years has been from our treatment of a passage in Romans that starts in the seventh chapter. The Apostle Paul wrote the following:

So I find this law at work: When I want to do good, evil is right there with me. For in my inner being I delight in God's law; but I see another law at work in the members of my body, waging war against the law of my mind and making me a prisoner of the law of sin at work within my members. What a wretched man I am! Who will rescue me from this body of death? Thanks be to God—through Jesus Christ our Lord! So then, I myself in my mind am a slave to God's law, but in the sinful nature a slave to the law of sin. Therefore, there is now no condemnation for those who are in Christ Jesus, because through Christ Jesus the law of the Spirit of life set me free from the law of sin and death. (Rom. 7:21–8:2)

This is where the typical sermon ends. Everyone thanks God because there is no condemnation for those in Christ. "Thank goodness," people say. "Praise God for Christ's blood!"

But take a closer look. That is *not* how this passage in Romans intended for you to use the blood of Christ. The very next crucial, but often left out, sentence reads:

For what the law was powerless to do in that it was weakened by the sinful nature, God did by sending his own Son in the likeness of sinful man to be a sin offering. And so he condemned sin in sinful man, in order that the righteous requirements of the law might be fully met in us, who do not live according to the sinful nature but according to the Spirit. Those who live according to the sinful nature have their minds set on what that nature desires; but those who live in accordance with the Spirit have their minds set on what the Spirit desires. The mind of sinful man is death, but the mind controlled by the Spirit is life and peace; the sinful mind is hostile to God. It does not submit to God's law, nor can it do so. Those controlled by the sinful nature cannot please God. You, however, are controlled not by the sinful nature but by the Spirit, if the Spirit of God lives in you. (Rom. 8:3–9a)

If you consider the section that describes our struggles in the context of the whole passage, you will see that Paul was *not* justifying staying in a sinful state but showing you how to be *set free* to sin no more. It starts with your mind, and your mind should be on what God wants. But if your mind is on what you want, then you are being controlled by the sinful nature.

To ask the Spirit of God to rule your spirit, you must set your will aside and be still. Ask God what He wants every day. Seeing, wanting, and grabbing are how we have been raised, but we must reverse that. There are many other religious groups whose members have been raised less selfishly than Christian children. Other religions teach their children that there are selfish or evil urges and that they also have a competing urge to do good. By the time a boy or girl turns twelve or thirteen—the age of accountability—those religions teach that the urge to do good should control every person. These individuals are taught in the early years that they do have a selfish nature, but it is not to be nurtured. Rather, looking to the needs of others is more important than gratifying this selfish nature. Selfishness is not tolerated in many Eastern religions—but for the wrong reason: just for peace on earth. At least this is a step in the right direction. From this passage, we can see that Christianity, however, is teaching that we are to please only one spirit and that is the spirit of Jesus Christ and God the Father—not mankind. After trying

> *After trying only to please God, you see that God has an ironic plan—a plan that will ultimately prosper you and take care of you faster and better than your own "take care of yourself" scheme.*

only to please God, you see that God has an ironic plan—a plan that will ultimately prosper you and take care of you faster and better than your own "take care of yourself" scheme. He is a genius.

Understand that having the spirit of Christ is also having an attitude or mind-set of Christ—a spirit that is willing to go to the cross. This passage from Romans 8—which clearly states that we are now free to leave our old desires and sins—goes on to say even more:

You, however, are controlled not by the sinful nature but by the Spirit, if the Spirit of God lives in you. And if anyone does not have the Spirit of Christ, he does not belong to Christ. But if Christ is in you, your body is dead because of sin, yet your spirit is alive because of righteousness. And if the Spirit of him who raised Jesus from the dead is living in you, he who raised Christ from the dead will also give life to your mortal bodies through his Spirit, who lives in you. Therefore, brothers, we have an obligation—but it is not to the sinful nature, to live according to it. For if you live according to the sinful nature, you will die; but if by the Spirit you put to death the misdeeds of the body, you will live, because those who are led by the Spirit of God are sons of God. For you did not receive a spirit that makes you a slave again to fear, but you received the Spirit of sonship. And by him we cry, "Abba, Father." The Spirit himself testifies with our spirit that we are God's children. Now if we are children, then we are heirs—heirs of God and co-heirs with Christ, if indeed we share in his sufferings in order that we may also share in his glory. (Rom. 8:9–17)

If you live daily asking God, "What do You want? You first. Your will first," then you will please God, and then He will come in and reward you by giving you something you want, and then He will take away your old desires so that it is not a battle anymore. You must not let yourself focus on what you want—just what God wants, pleasing Him and looking for the rewards from Him. Also, make yourself highly aware of how horrible a separation from God would be, because if you live according to the sinful nature, you will die. You will die a physical as well as a spiritual death. You will no longer have God as your ally and your comfort, nor will you have the life that goes along with it. If you sit down long enough to understand spiritual life and spiritual death, you will make the right choice when you are tried and tested. If you do not like the choices you have been making, recognize that they have been *your* wants and *your* will, and then repent. Tear yourself away and obey God. Give Him your attention and look to Him to fill your needs and wants, and you will live (read Ezek. 18).

All along, Scripture has clearly pointed out that we must rise above by focusing on heavenly things. Galatians 6:7–8 tells us that God cannot be mocked, but that a man reaps what he sows. If he sows to please his sinful nature, from that nature he will reap destruction. But if he sows to please the Spirit, from that nature he will reap eternal life. Make sure that you take these passages to heart because Satan's biggest lie of all is that God does not care about one more binge of food or one more moment spent deeply desiring another person who is not your spouse or one more magnetic spending spree—He does care. He cares very much because He wants a pure New Jerusalem—a holy group magnetized to Him (1 Peter 2:9). You cannot be devoted to God and be constantly and daily devoted to the refrigerator, the alcohol, or an affair at the same time.

God's mercies are new every morning, and He is waiting for us all to come home. But He will not indulge us if we are like the prodigal son in Luke 15. God is not going to run to the pigpen and pull us out.

God is not going to run to the pigpen and pull us out. He is not going to deliver hamburgers to the pigpen.

He is not going to deliver hamburgers to the pigpen. The prodigal son looked for happiness and life in the world—only to find that the world took his money and gave him nothing back but scraps for pigs. God is now waiting for us to climb out of the pigpen and walk home. When we come home we will get the fatted calf (I always love to point out that even God serves red meat), the robe, and the ring. To come home, we need to focus on the Father, stay in His Word, listen to and read the toughest and most challenging lessons and sermons—not the ones that sweetly preach, "You're too hard on yourself" and "God loves you just the way you are." That's the kiss of Judas—the betrayal of the life of Jesus.

The major lesson you have learned is that God is not asking you just to quit smoking, drinking, overeating, or gambling. God is giving you another avenue through which to vent your passion: Himself and Jesus Christ. Go to God through Jesus Christ, and watch His good, personal, loving touch fill you better than any binge or spree or indulgence you have ever had.

SECRET OF THE PRISON

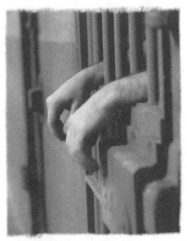

So what is the secret of this prison you are in? It is that you have walked into your prison by your own free will. You are holding on to the prison bars—they are not holding you. You are embracing your prison or stronghold. Your stronghold does not care about you. Do you see that your fingers are holding tight to this refrigerator door and prison pantry, and there are no armed guards forcing you and keeping you in? There are no keys that keep you locked up. Satan was defeated when Jesus walked the path to the heart of the Father and willingly accepted death on a cross for our sins. Isaiah 61:1b states, "He has sent me to bind up the brokenhearted, to proclaim freedom for the captives and release from darkness for the prisoners." The prison doors are open!

Do you want to walk out today? Then let go of the food. Let it go. You can do it. Food will never love you back. Escape and walk away.

Take your hands off the prison bars, and stop reading the graffiti written all over the walls. You are free, my friends, to walk out right in front of the masses that want to hold on to all the comfortable but self-destructive lies. Let go of the prison bars (food) and hold to the tough but liberating teachings of Jesus Christ—*the Cross*. As you walk away, open your eyes, and see God facing you and then taking your hands and pulling you away from the prison and toward Himself. Everywhere you go, imagine yourself arm in arm with your best Friend, God Almighty. You have not merely let go; you have let go to get something greater back! From this day forward, your life is going to be radically different because you now know the Secret of the Prison: the doors are unlocked and the prison gate is open. The remaining prisoners are there behind the walls of fat by their *own free will*—it is their *choice* of worship. Let go and join the escaped prisoners who no longer listen to the lies of the people who never want to stop kissing the food!

Jesus said, "If you hold to my teaching, you are really my disciples. Then you will know the truth, and the truth will set you free." (John 8:31b–32)

What You Can Do Today

➤ *Go where God is leading you in Scripture.*

➤ *Seek the truth.* When you hear a prison lie that is very tempting to believe, search out the truth in God's Word, and look to Him for your guidance, not to the lie. Know that there is only *one truth.* Reference the following passages so that you can get a clearer understanding of this concept: John 18:37; John 16:13; John 17:17; 2 Timothy 2:22–26; Galatians 2:4–5; John 4:23–24; John 3:19–21; John 8:31–32.

➤ *Notice God's gifts.* When you begin to feel defeated, stop and take note of all the time and attention God is giving to you. He is fighting very hard for your devotion—how can you think that you are unlovely or unwanted?

➤ *Review the foundational principles of The Weigh Down Workshop[†] in Appendix A and Appendix B.* Starting right now, *commit* yourself to focus on God and His will every time you find yourself wanting to eat when your body is not calling for food.

➤ *Ask for God's help.* Whenever you feel yourself struggling, stop and ask God, "God, what do *You* want for me today? I want to do *Your* will." Your battles will subside as God removes your old desires and replaces them with His Spirit.

➤ *Compare the "old you" to the "new you."* Make a list that compares your old prison ways to all the wonderful ways that God is setting your heart free as you walk away from the prison. You will be amazed at the things He has already done!

_____

_____

_____

_____

The Tiny Units of Chocolate

When you eat chocolate, it is a good idea to start with small amounts in order to savor every bite and every morsel. In my past, I have been known to eat a king-size candy bar in one, two, or three bites without ever truly tasting it. Now, it takes me two to four (or more!) bites to eat a *miniature* candy bar, and I enjoy every tasty bit! Not only that, but when I eat a regular-size chocolate-covered peppermint candy, I will break it up into several tiny pieces. This way, I can savor each piece as I let it melt in my mouth. First, I can taste the chocolate by itself, and then I can taste the creamy center as it melts into a fresh mint flavor. Another favorite is any combination candy bar that comes with layers of chocolate, caramel, nuts, or a crispy cookie or nougat center. I will eat the overlapping chocolate edges first before I begin eating the actual candy bar. Once all of the edges have been eaten, I will then begin to eat the candy bar layer by layer. First, I eat the chocolate on top, then work my way through the caramel. As I work toward the crispy center, many times I find that there is still another layer of chocolate or caramel underneath, depending on the candy bar. What used to take me only a second or two to eat can now take me up to twenty minutes or more—and the really nice thing is that I usually have some of the candy bar left

Just because it is small doesn't mean you have to pop the whole thing in your mouth. You now have a new definition of **small**.

over for another time! My office drawer is full of chocolate, but to be honest, now I get much more enjoyment from giving it away rather than eating it myself.

seven

BACKSTROKING THE RED SEA

When we read about the plagues in chapter 3, we discovered they were really battles for our hearts—battles between God and Egypt. What we learned is that even though God has made Himself invisible—and that would be analogous to tying His right hand behind His back in a fight—He was still able to definitively beat the competition to an unrecognizable pulp.

THE RESCUE

God has done His homework. He has shown us His passionate, jealous love, and He has shown us that He is not going to sit still and let the competition steal our hearts away. God has shown us that He is going to rescue and save us and make a distinction between those who have a heart for Him and those who have a heart for Egypt. God's awesome victory showed that He was the God of all gods, and the Israelites' hearts were drawn to follow this mighty Warrior to the desert! So God won the first showdown with Pharaoh. Satan knows he is no competition face-to-face. Now that God has helped us see the light of day when it comes to Egypt, Satan has to use something more discreet to fool us—clouding the mind by using the lie.

The Desert Honeymoon

When God saved us from Egypt and brought us across the Red Sea and into the desert, we had such a honeymoon. There were singing and dancing on the other side of finding out how God saved us from having to love the food and enabled us to love Him. Those first couple of weeks, every time we wanted to run to the food, we ran to God and focused on Him. So, we lost some weight right away, even while we were enjoying small amounts of chocolate and pizza and hamburgers—after years of denying ourselves these treats. We were floating on the freedom of not worrying about food and focusing on food anymore. We were in prayer constantly, thanking God for His program and for showing us the true way to eat. But as time went by, some of us might have found ourselves plateaued on the scale. The next thing we knew, we hadn't lost weight for weeks, or months, maybe even years.

We were in prayer constantly, thanking God for His program and for showing us the true way to eat. But as time went by, some of us might have found ourselves plateaued on the scale.

You have thought that since you have plateaued and you are feeling pain again after the honeymoon, it must be the heat of the desert. You say, "Oh, it's just one of those desert storms. God is just working on me. I'm waiting on the Lord. He is working on something else in my life right now. He will complete the work He started." Yes, you do struggle in the desert, but the struggles in the desert are the pain and the suffering from obedience, not the pain that comes from hugging the refrigerator and trying to get God to repent or change His mind so that you can have two masters. The pain of obedience is the suffering that comes from dying to your will—letting go of what your flesh really wants in favor of what God wants. It means going without and waiting on God instead of grabbing for instant gratification. It means giving up all your self-serving and self-promoting plans in favor of God's plan for your life. The suffering of obedience is short-lived because it doesn't take long to realize that God's rewards for obedience far outweigh anything you have given up to follow Him. This suffering is not the pain of disobedience! Remember, those who were disobedient died in the desert.

THE BACKSTROKE

No, if we find ourselves in the pantry and refrigerator night after night, we are still in the arms of Egypt. But I'm afraid the deceiver has told us that we have made God our choice and that we have left Egypt! So even after the mighty exodus, many of us have slowly done the backstroke across the Red Sea and wound up back on the shoreline of Egypt. We are actually back in Egypt, but Pharaoh or Satan has redecorated Egypt now that we have returned, so that we will not recognize it. Where once there were pyramids, there are now church pews and stained-glass windows. It's a new and improved Egypt that's more encompassing. Now, the slaves are on the church pew, but they have to make enough space on this pew for their ball-and-chain and their lover. For some, it is enough space for a refrigerator; for others, it is a safe full of money. Another church member drags in a medicine cabinet, and still others are chained to a cooler of six-packs. Some chests are bigger than others. The person chained to a chest full of pride takes up a whole pew. Some prisoners hide on the back pews or in the balcony with a closet full of secret sins. If you ever confront them, it's like opening up Pandora's box; you might release a few demons to roam freely around the pews, seeking places to enter.

It's a twisted Egypt, with sermons that allow you to love what you want to on this earth and thank God each week for His repentance, that is, for taking back His rules and commands and allowing us to continue to indulge ourselves. And of course, we thank Him for Jesus Christ, who has made the three-way love affair possible (you and God and your food) by granting all-encompassing forgiveness. It's a new Egypt that has sermons centering on the fact that it is wrong to feel guilt after you have come to the Lord. They cry out, "Drop your guilt—that is from Satan! Satan is the accuser of the brethren. We should claim our status as sons!" But you cannot be a prodigal son and an at-home son at the same time. The prodigal son sits on the pew week after week, wondering where the fatted calf is, and his faith weakens as his unanswered prayers multiply.

It's a contorted world where we rarely hear sermons that condemn loving the food and enjoying God. Well, I am here to tell you the truth: we cannot love the food and enjoy God. We should be loving God and enjoying the food. When we seek God first, a relationship is birthed. But God pulls back from the heart of the one who chooses other gods to adore. How could we ever put God in second place? My friends, it's one thing to be caught red-handed one time with another lover, but many of us are repeatedly choosing to secretly embrace something else on this earth. We even bring it into the only place in the world that is not supposed to have the world in it—the only place on earth where God asks for it to be just Him.

You see, God has allowed the entire earth to be under the control of Satan. That's more than fair, don't you agree? Can't we allow just one sanctuary where God has our full attention without any competition for our hearts? Oh, no, we've brought the world into the church, which is our hearts. It is unbearable to think about how painful and how insulting this is to God, yet how entertaining this is to Satan. On top of this, we call this perverted Egypt the "New Jerusalem" or the "called out" or the "church," confusing the world around us. Pharaoh has discreetly climbed back in the driver's seat, and we are enslaved all over again.

I hear so many people claim that their six- to twelve-month plateau in weight loss is the desert. But think with me . . . if we call this a desert, then it is a swamp, an undertow, quicksand. And we're worse off than we were before because we've labeled this delusion as a more progressive part of the journey of salvation instead of a retreat. We have concocted such a defeated desert scene that young sojourners would never want to follow in our footsteps.

The Largest Delusion

People do not know up from down. This fact is seen clearly in Micah 3:1–5:

> "Listen, you leaders of Jacob, you rulers of the house of Israel. Should you not know justice, you who hate good and love evil; who tear the skin from my people and the flesh from their bones; who eat my people's flesh, strip off their skin and break their bones in pieces; who chop them up like meat for the pan, like flesh for the pot?" Then they will cry out to the LORD, but he will not answer them. At that time he will hide his face from them because of the evil they have done. This is what the LORD says: "As for the prophets who lead my people astray, if one feeds them, they proclaim 'peace'; if he does not, they prepare to wage war against him."

When you are following an idol or a false leader and you don't know your own way, you could be traveling east when you want to go west. You could be headed toward Egypt and slavery with the food when you actually want to go to the desert where God is.

This false status is no small matter. I see it as the largest delusion of the body of Christ—an invisible, undetectable cancer that has permeated every denomination. So that instead of a healthy, athletic, powerful, and magnetic body of Christ, it is a sad, sickly, cancerous body of Christ lying on a hospital bed with an IV bag. We lie on the hospital bed, devising evangelical church programs to invite the world into this "saved" state, and yet we can't even get up and walk. This is hardly an evangelical state for the body of Christ. Who wants this? Week after week, people sit on the church pew, enslaved, and claim, "I'm saved! I'm saved!" And yet their necks are strangled by a ball-and-chain, and they wonder why they can't drink in the Water of Life, and they wonder why they are thirsty even though they are supposedly sitting in the middle of an oasis.

How do you know if your heart has drifted back to Egypt? If the thought of not getting to your food panics you or leaves you with an empty feeling, then you have an idol. If you catch yourself thinking about food or money or sex all throughout the day, that is where your heart is. If talking about God is awkward, then God can't be your hero. I'm not talking about discussing church activities or church members (gossip); I'm referring to getting excited when you find somebody else who will talk to you about God's character and your answered prayers. So, how can you tell if you are chained and enslaved to an idol? If you are praying to God to get rid of it, you have got it. If you find yourself, night after night, evening after evening, hanging around the kitchen and bingeing after everyone else has gone to bed, something's wrong.

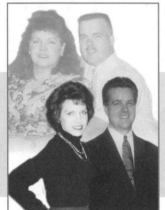

My husband has lost 60 pounds, and I've lost 140 pounds. We've both kept our weight off for three years. Not only has God rescued us from bondage to overeating, but He has changed our hearts and saved our marriage. We would not be married right now if we had not gone through this program and learned obedience to God.
Jeff & Gina Graves—Murfreesboro, TN

Surrendering to God in matters of food led Jeff and Gina to surrender their marriage to Him as well.

FOOD GOD VS. THE TRUE GOD

We have learned that Egypt is no match for God. The story of the devastating plagues has great symbolism. Food cannot save us. Has food clothed us? As we have said before, no. It has robbed us of our clothing. In fact, just finding clothing that fits is a major ordeal. Has food helped us with our self-esteem? To the contrary, it has left us depleted of self-esteem. We are more timid, fearful, and prone to panic attack disorders. Has food helped us with our relationships at work or at home? Only if we are fooling ourselves and think that we are fooling our loved ones. No, if you were to ask your family about the pain they have endured because your heart was in love with food, you might get an earful. Has loving food or worshiping food helped you, encouraged you, or given back to you anything? Anything? No—it is an emptiness and a darkness that have robbed your soul so deeply that you don't have words to describe it, except death. It is the ultimate unrequited love. Food cannot love you back. I'm basically exposing food for what it is. Food is a false help, a false comfort, a false entertainment, and a false friend. In other words, it is a false god.

In sharp contrast, you can prove that our God is a God and the only God. When you give ten minutes of your heart to God, He multiplies that amount and gives you back an hour. When you hand over ten dollars to the Father, He generates one hundred dollars' worth of blessings. When you give Him just some of your strength and your soul, it propagates life and health inside your heart. Sometimes when you least expect it, He lavishes you with generosity. And there is nothing like those quick answered prayers that make you feel as if you have just whispered your wishes to your best friend.

Have we forgotten what a God is? A God—a true God—doesn't need anything. If He did, He wouldn't be a God. Jehovah doesn't need your ten minutes or even your twenty-four hours. He doesn't need your twenty dollars. God doesn't need your heart or your soul or your mind. That's why He can give it back to you, plus some. He is the Source of time, and He is the Source of love. He is the Supplier of gold, and He is the Creator of food. He is the Fountain of life. Yes, I have experienced this truth. He is the Alpha, and He is the Omega. He is the Beginning, and He is the End. He is the only Source—find me another. Try giving your heart to football, baseball, basketball, or hockey. As you adore the athletes, the irony is that many times you become a couch potato, somehow full of anger. Try making your spouse a god, and you will run him off. Your spouse is your helpmate, not your god. Just try giving your heart to money, and you'll find

God doesn't need your heart or your soul or your mind. That's why He can give it back to you, plus some.

yourself in poverty. Try giving yourself to sexual lust, and you'll find yourself divorced, lonely, or diseased. You could even adore the activities surrounding church and not be worshiping God. The heart is deceitful above all things. Churchgoers have made all kinds of things a "legal" god, such as "their" singing, "their" ministry, and "their"

flock because their god is the praise of man, but down deep they cannot submit to the one, true God where He asks them to. *The* God is not their god. Find me another true god—you can't. There's only one. He is the only choice. Yes, our churches have made Him one of the choices, but not *the* Choice.

EXCHANGING GODS

We go to the church building each week and give lip service, but we have changed gods. We have exchanged gods. What has God done that we have exchanged Him for food?

Our heavenly Father has lived through this before. Israel tried to maintain its status as Israel—God's beloved—while chasing after things to make it feel good, comfort it, and advance it—a job only God could do. One such description of Israel's wayward heart is in Jeremiah:

> The word of the LORD came to me: "Go and proclaim in the hearing of Jerusalem: 'I remember the devotion of your youth, how as a bride you loved me and followed me through the desert, through a land not sown. Israel was holy to the LORD, the firstfruits of his harvest; all

who *devoured her were held guilty, and disaster overtook them,'"* declares the LORD. . . . *"What fault did your fathers find in me, that they strayed so far from me? They followed worthless idols and became worthless themselves. They did not ask, 'Where is the LORD, who brought us up out of Egypt and led us through the barren wilderness, through a land of deserts and rifts, a land of drought and darkness, a land where no one travels and no one lives?' I brought you into a fertile land to eat its fruit and rich produce. But you came and defiled my land and made my inheritance detestable.*

"The priests did not ask, 'Where is the LORD?' Those who deal with the law did not know me; the leaders rebelled against me. The prophets prophesied by Baal, following worthless idols. Therefore I bring charges against you again," declares the LORD. *"And I will bring charges against your children's children. Cross over to the coasts of Kittim and look, send to Kedar and observe closely; see if there has ever been anything like this: Has a nation ever changed its gods? (Yet they are not gods at all.) But my people have exchanged their Glory for worthless idols. Be appalled at this, O heavens, and shudder with great horror,"* declares the LORD. *"My people have committed two sins: They have forsaken me, the spring of living water, and have dug their own cisterns, broken cisterns that cannot hold water. Is Israel a servant, a slave by birth? Why then has he become plunder? Lions have roared; they have growled at him. They have laid waste his land; his towns are burned and deserted. Also, the men of Memphis and Tahpanhes have shaved the crown of your head.*

"Have you not brought this on yourselves by forsaking the LORD your God when he led you in the way? Now why go to Egypt to drink water from the Shihor? And why go to Assyria to drink water from the River? Your wickedness will punish you; your backsliding will rebuke you. Consider then and realize how evil and bitter it is for you when you forsake the LORD your God and have no awe of me," declares the LORD, the LORD Almighty. *"Long ago you broke off your yoke and tore off your bonds; you said, 'I will not serve you!' Indeed, on every high hill and under every spreading tree you lay down as a prostitute. I*

had planted you like a choice vine of sound and reliable stock. How then did you turn against me into a corrupt, wild vine? Although you wash yourself with soda and use an abundance of soap, the stain of your guilt is still before me," declares the Sovereign LORD.

"How can you say, 'I am not defiled; I have not run after the Baals'? See how you behaved in the valley; consider what you have done. You are a swift she-camel running here and there, a wild donkey accustomed to the desert, sniffing the wind in her craving—in her heat who can restrain her? Any males that pursue her need not tire themselves; at mating time they will find her. . . . But you said, 'It's no use! I love foreign gods, and I must go after them.'

"As a thief is disgraced when he is caught, so the house of Israel is disgraced—they, their kings and their officials, their priests and their prophets. They say to wood, 'You are my father,' and to stone, 'You gave me birth.' They have turned their backs to me and not their faces; yet when they are in trouble, they say, 'Come and save us!' Where then are the gods you made for yourselves? Let them come if they can save you when you are in trouble! For you have as many gods as you have towns, O Judah. Why do you bring charges against me? You have all rebelled against me," declares the LORD.

"In vain I punished your people; they did not respond to correction. Your sword has devoured your prophets like a ravening lion. You of this generation, consider the word of the LORD: *"Have I been a desert to Israel or a land of great darkness? Why do my people say, 'We are free to roam; we will come to you no more'?*

"Does a maiden forget her jewelry, a bride her wedding ornaments? Yet my people have forgotten me, days without number. How skilled you are at pursuing love! Even the worst of women can learn from your ways. . . . Yet in spite of all this you say, 'I am innocent; he is not angry with me.' But I will pass judgment on you because you say, 'I have not sinned.'

"Why do you go about so much, changing your ways? You will be disappointed by Egypt as you were by Assyria. You will also leave

that place with your hands on your head, for the LORD has rejected
those you trust; you will not be helped by them.

"If a man divorces his wife and she leaves him and marries another
man, should he return to her again? Would not the land be completely
defiled? But you have lived as a prostitute with many lovers—would
you now return to me?" declares the LORD. "Look up to the barren
heights and see. Is there any place where you have not been ravished?
By the roadside you sat waiting for lovers, sat like a nomad in the
desert. You have defiled the land with your prostitution and wicked-
ness. Therefore the showers have been withheld, and no spring rains
have fallen. Yet you have the brazen look of a prostitute; you refuse to
blush with shame. Have you not just called to me: 'My Father, my
friend from my youth, will you always be angry? Will your wrath con-
tinue forever?' This is how you talk, but you do all the evil you can."
(Jer. 2:1–3:5)

This passage describes exactly how I see many of the church buildings today—the groups of people called to honor Him. All other
groups on earth have their gods, and yet the one group called to serve
the God has casually exchanged *the* God for the food god and the god
of self and other worldly idols. God will hold the pastors, teachers,
elders, and deacons of the churches to greater responsibility if they
have allowed idols.

But the sheep are in bad shape partially because of their lack of
awareness of false prophets—the counterfeit pastors and preachers.
Sheep are made to follow. That's why sheep must take their time in
examining shepherds or leaders. False shepherds make feeble or little
effort in inspiring you to turn from sin. However, they make much
ado about how God loves you just the way you are, and they encourage you to depend upon a false relationship—one that Jesus and God
never allowed. Jesus said, "Go now and leave your life of sin" (John
8:11b).

And look at God's words in these passages from Ezekiel 18:

What do you people mean by quoting this proverb about the land of Israel: "The fathers eat sour grapes, and the children's teeth are set on edge"? As surely as I live, declares the Sovereign LORD, you will no longer quote this proverb in Israel. For every living soul belongs to me, the father as well as the son—both alike belong to me. The soul who sins is the one who will die. (vv. 2–4)

The righteousness of the righteous man will be credited to him, and the wickedness of the wicked will be charged against him. But if a wicked man turns away from all the sins he has committed and keeps all my decrees and does what is just and right, he will surely live; he will not die. None of the offenses he has committed will be remembered against him. Because of the righteous things he has done, he will live. Do I take any pleasure in the death of the wicked? declares the Sovereign LORD. Rather, am I not pleased when they turn from their ways and live? But if a righteous man turns from his righteousness and commits sin and does the same detestable things the wicked man does, will he live? None of the righteous things he has done will be remembered. Because of the unfaithfulness he is guilty of and because of the sins he has committed, he will die. (vv. 20b–24)

Reading all of Ezekiel 18 will make this idea of leaving sin even clearer to you.

False shepherds and false prophets look like the real bill, and it takes great discernment to see that they are counterfeit bills and not genuine articles. It is hard to see the heart, but once you do, you see a very different motive deep down. In other words, false prophets will look and sound like true prophets, with a hard-to-detect difference. False prophets have always been more abundant than God's true prophets. Prophets who are willing to tell the truth and have no desire to tickle the ears of the people are true prophets. In 1 Kings, we see that when Elijah represented God, he stood against 450 false prophets. When Micaiah prophesied against King Ahab, Ahab called in 400 false prophets—and these were Israel's prophets: 1 against 400. The 400 prophesied that the Lord was with Ahab. In Jeremiah, we are warned against lying prophets:

They fill you with false hopes. They speak visions from their own minds, not from the mouth of the LORD. They keep saying to those who despise me, "The LORD says: You will have peace." And to all who follow the stubbornness of their hearts they say, "No harm will come to you." (Jer. 23:16–17)

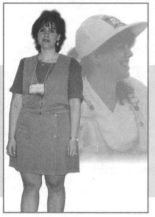

I feel like I was involved with "super mega Christian woman syndrome." With four small children, I was involved in preschool, sports, carpooling, my Bible studies, and Christian women's club. My life was full of so many "good things," how could I possibly give them up? But I now know how to live a life of full peace and joy!
Tonya Cardente—Sacramento, CA

Tonya Cardente now lets God organize her time rather than trying to do it all herself.

Jesus warns us again and again to be on our guard against those who tickle our ears. Jesus said, "And if your eye causes you to sin, pluck it out. It is better for you to enter the kingdom of God with one eye than to have two eyes and be thrown into hell" (Mark 9:47). This is a tough but clear calling to sell everything and invest in this kingdom and holy priesthood.

So the warning is to the religious, to the churchgoers, to God's people, to be careful not to surround yourself with teachings that use the blood of Christ to allow you to have two lovers. Jesus' blood was never intended to leave you in Egypt. It was never intended to be used to bring Egypt into the desert, either, which is what we have done to God's church. "If the Son sets you free, you will be free indeed" (John 8:36). First John 5 tells us: "This is love for God: to obey his commands. And his commands are not burdensome, for everyone born of God overcomes the world" (vv. 3–4a). The blood and life of Christ are not only for the forgiveness of past sins and stumbling sins, but the power to help you get out of continual sins.

RELIGIOUS ACTIVITIES VS. PURE WHOLEHEARTED LOVE AND DEVOTION

Another lesson from Israel's history is that if we get too busy doing religious things, we might look up and discover that our hearts are not where they should be. We might like going to church services because we just happen to enjoy the fellowship; we just love making pies for the sick members of the congregation because we love cooking; we love heading up church projects because we naturally love to organize; we come to every service because we just love being a part of this group. We sing in the church choir just because we love to sing. We've been deceived by "playing church." We do what is natural for the body of Christ—but our lips can sing about God while our hearts still reside in serving the food or other secret sins.

Likewise, we can look up in the middle of a Weigh Down† class—which is really just a gathering of "the called out" who study God's Word and practice repentance—and find ourselves gaining weight. Ironically, we are growing in a relationship with food, and this is in a fellowship provided by God where we are supposed to be growing away from this relationship with food. We can meet with the group assembled each week and confess the food we overate. No, really, sometimes we make light of the overeating of the week. And then we use meeting time to justify one another's overeating. We can attend Weigh Down† and love it. We love the videos; we love the Bible study; we share our excitement with our coworkers and families, but we don't give the high places to God, and so session after session we don't lose the weight. You may think you have left Egypt because you have listened to God's Word on the tapes or read the Bible or enjoyed the fellowship.

There are people who have lost all their weight by sitting in Weigh Down† Bible classes and reading the Word of God, but their hearts remained in love with food. They failed to give their hearts to God, and so they gained their weight back. Try to be honest about where your heart is—whether it is still wanting to hold on to this earth or wanting to cling to the Father. Because, my friends, that's the key.

Don't you see? We can look religious, we can be religious, we can be around religious activities and enjoy God and other churchgoing people, yet not love Him or wholeheartedly obey Him. If we're not losing weight, it's possible that we are secretly kissing the food. It's a heart problem—our hearts are still not in the right place. Isaiah 29:13 tells us that "the Lord says: 'These people come near to me with their mouth and honor me with their lips, but their hearts are far from me.'" We need to make it a priority to know where our hearts are, just as we want to know where our children are at night.

Next, we need to be aware that Satan is a big fat liar, and that he will always tell us that we are somewhere when we are not. To make a dent in this overwhelming delusion brought upon God's people, let's learn about Satan's lies and get away from false prophets who make us feel safe while we are still in love with the world (Jer. 23:16–18; Lam. 2:14; Ezek. 22:23–28; Matt. 7:15).

Satan could tell you that you are saved from loving the world. Satan says, "You don't love the world. You love God." False prophets back him up and tell you that you are in God's favor and abiding in Christ while you privately kiss the food. If the human heart is so easily deceived, then you of all people should be most mindful, careful, watchful, leery, observant, open-eyed, conscientious, and cautious—being able to identify exactly the treasures of your heart because, as it says in Matthew 6:21, "where your treasure is, there your heart will be also." Many times your children reflect what you adore, and this helps you realize the truth and the truth sets you free.

LOVING GOD AND LOVING FOOD

What if our hearts are divided: we love God *and* we love food? Well, my friends, it is simply impossible. You see, the Bible teaches us that we cannot have two masters. Matthew 6:24 states, "No one can serve two masters. Either he will hate the one and love the other, or he will be devoted to the one and despise the other. You cannot serve both God and Money." Likewise, you cannot serve both God and food. Are you obeying God, who says not to be greedy with food, or are you obeying the food that says, "Come and eat me"? You are either losing weight or not losing weight. This lets you know whom you obey. The one you obey is your master. You are serving *the* God or the food god.

You were born to love, you were born to worship, you were born to serve, but you cannot love, worship, and serve two things at one time. It's impossible. Even if you want to, you cannot. God ingeniously programmed both of these unique phenomena of the human heart: you were born to love (in fact, you are loving something even as you read this), but you cannot love two things at one time. Don't listen to that lie of Satan.

Practically all the different authors of the Bible brought up this major precept of God. Jesus pointed out that there are two gates— one is wide that leads to destruction, and one is narrow that leads to life. In Joshua 24, Joshua made it clear that there were only two choices:

> *Now fear the LORD and serve him with all faithfulness. Throw away the gods your forefathers worshiped beyond the River and in Egypt, and serve the LORD. But if serving the LORD seems undesirable to you, then choose for yourselves this day whom you will serve, whether the gods your forefathers served beyond the River, or the gods of the Amorites, in whose land you are living. But as for me and my household, we will serve the LORD. (Josh. 24:14–15)*

Moses cried out in Deuteronomy 30 that there were only two choices: life and death. Ezekiel pointed out that there were only two choices: righteousness and unrighteousness. The writer of Hebrews made sure that we understood that there were only two categories: the obedient and the disobedient, the believer and the unbeliever. And the Apostle John wrote of only two types of people: those who love and those who hate. There are only two destinations: heaven and hell. And finally, God Himself gave us two choices in Exodus 20: love Him or hate Him. Never, in any of these categories, is there even the slightest hint of a gray zone—an uncommitted, unattached, or lukewarm option. There is no middle ground. Whether you like it or not, you are in one or the other.

Never, in any of these categories, is there even the slightest hint of a gray zone—an uncommitted, unattached, or lukewarm option. There is no middle ground. Whether you like it or not, you are in one or the other.

We read in 1 John: "Do not love the world or anything in the world. If anyone loves the world, the love of the Father is not in him" (2:15). Throughout the Old and New Testaments, God gets upset at His children for even turning to another lover, much less trying to talk Him into letting all three into the same relationship! That is analogous to asking your spouse to allow you to have a second lover in bed with him! This is *unthinkable,* especially to such a wonderful God.

How to Swim Back to the Desert

What can you do now? Stop asking God to repent. Stop begging Him to change His commands and His boundaries. Stop asking for His blessings while you refuse to obey His will. God has made no provisions to allow you to have devotion both ways, but has made every provision for you to make a choice one way or the other.

Confess. Be honest and confess to God where your heart is. If it is back in Egypt, admit it; then simply turn your entire heart to God Almighty. Our God is so great that even if our hearts have been misplaced, we can—with a sincere, heartfelt focus—walk back again on dry land to the sweet desert sand. And the neat thing is that the longer you stay in the desert, the more you fall in love with God. And the more you fall in love with God, the less likely it becomes that you will ever flirt with Egypt again. It's all a matter of the heart. So you want to work on keeping your heart in the desert long enough to become deeply rooted in the love of God and no longer divided.

Be assured that you can return to God or transfer your love to God. We see this in Jeremiah 3:

> *"Return, faithless Israel," declares the LORD, "I will frown on you no longer, for I am merciful," declares the LORD, "I will not be angry forever. Only acknowledge your guilt—you have rebelled against the LORD your God, you have scattered your favors to foreign gods under every spreading tree, and have not obeyed me," declares the LORD. "Return, faithless people," declares the LORD, "for I am your husband."* (vv. 12b–14a)

Even if we have developed a heart-pounding crush on food—where we dress for the food in our stretch clothes, we plan secret rendezvous with the food late at night, we hear the voice of the one we love, and thinking of food is even what gets us out of bed in the morning—moving from Egypt to the desert is as easy as when you had a crush on some guy in high school. You loved that person. But when the new guy walked in, you no longer even wanted the old one to call your name. You didn't want him to write you notes or phone you, and you even avoided walking down the hallway where his locker was. The old lover became repulsive; that's how it is with food for me now. I don't want my old love *food* to call my name unless I'm hungry. And just as a little-bitty rudder can change the direction of a ship, your heart was made to turn around. The simple tool used to move the rudder is called "choice." If I ever feel my heart beginning to wander, I find something God has made, such as flowers, and I marvel at Him again. When you choose today whom you will serve and focus on, your heart will follow. It's automatic. And you find your heart and mind back on the Father, where they belong.

I also remember that I am extremely blessed to have a chance to be alive at all, with a heart that beats. What are the odds of my DNA combination being in existence? And on top of that, I have the opportunity to show God that I love Him and appreciate this life by resisting temptation.

Just as God programmed you to love something—and you will automatically love something—God has programmed you to be able to transfer lovers today.

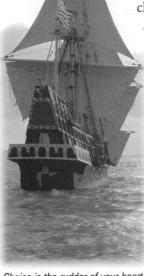

Choice is the rudder of your heart.

Don't ever worry that you will not be able to accomplish this transfer. You don't have to work on loving—you were born to love, like a bird was born to fly in the air. Look at how much of your mind and soul you have given to food—you are a good lover; you are familiar with intimacy. Likewise, you don't have to work on being able to transfer your devotion—you were born with the ability to transfer your devotion. Your only job description will be to concentrate on this hour-by-hour choice of adoration—this focus of adoration. And God is the right choice.

Remember, we fall in love with what we focus on. That's how we got into Egypt to start with, and that's how we're going to get out today. And as I've said before, that's how your children fall in love with cartoon action figures, rock stars, or sports figures. It's how a hero is birthed in your heart.

So, we're going to have to take this focus off the food. We must leave dieting and diet pills far behind us. Instead of focusing on the labels of the food, we need to start reading the labels of our hearts, and God's Word, and the labels of what God would want us to read. Know the statistics about Him. Know all the players—Abraham, Isaac, David, Jesus—and how they were all in love with God. Put His Scripture on the wall. Sing songs about Him. Write love notes to Him. Make sure you stay in His Word, so that you can know all the ins and outs about Him and what He wants; about Jesus, His wonderful Spirit, and His kingdom. That's focus.

The people who crossed the Red Sea made a choice of focus. They made a choice to serve the God who could send devastating plagues to Egypt but graceful protection to Goshen, the land inhabited by the Israelites. By their focus on the plagues and the favor God gave them, it was easy for them to make the right choice. Once they made the choice, they found themselves in the desert. What a world of grace we have at our fingertips! What a proposal we have from the God of the universe! It's called choice. It's a once-in-a-lifetime opportunity. We must sell everything that we are attached to so that we might obtain it. We must be like the merchant Jesus spoke of in Matthew 13:45–46: "Again, the kingdom of heaven is like a merchant looking for fine pearls. When he found one of great value, he went away and sold everything he had and bought it."

As you are making this choice to leave Egypt and follow God on dry land into the desert, remember what happened to the Israelites:

As Pharaoh approached, the Israelites looked up, and there were the Egyptians, marching after them. They were terrified and cried out to the LORD. They said to Moses, "Was it because there were no graves in Egypt that you have brought us to the desert to die? What have you done to us by bringing us out of Egypt? Didn't we say to you in Egypt, 'Leave us alone; let us serve the Egyptians'? It would have been better for us to serve the Egyptians than to die in the desert!" Moses

answered the people, "Do not be afraid. Stand firm and you will see
the deliverance the LORD will bring you today. The Egyptians you see
today you will never see again. The LORD will fight for you; you need
only to be still." Then the LORD said to Moses, "Why are you crying
out to me? Tell the Israelites to move on." (Ex. 14:10–15)

God told the Israelites to stand still, and then He told them to
move on. But if you study the passage a little more closely, when it
comes to the Egyptians, you need only to be still. Quit worrying
about Egypt and the Egyptians and Satan, for as God said, you will
never see them again. If you are spending your energy living in fear
of the attacks of Satan, then you are not focused on God. You can't
be in both camps. If you want to truly get out of Egypt and go into
the desert, what do you need to do? You need to move on! Get going!
Pursue God with all your might.

What does it mean to make this choice? Does it mean getting up in
the morning, choosing God, and then in the evening embracing the
food? No—the person doing these things is uncommitted to God.
Likewise, a person dependent upon worldly methods or man-made
rules could be sinking in the middle of the Red Sea. If this were your
spouse, you could call him a false, unfaithful, cheating, disloyal, adulterous spouse. A six-month plateau is a heart that could be trying to
entertain two lovers—but I promise that if your heart is divided, the
worldly lover will take over. Making this choice means you will be
saying no to food, and the desert sufferings you experience in dying
to self will be short-lived and rapidly rewarded with favor from God
and with weight loss. People making this choice will experience abundant love, joy, and peace. Would your spouse let you wander next
door every night? No—he would leave you! What makes you think
that God is going to let you wander down the steps and into the
kitchen every day for a secret rendezvous with food? God is not a
wimpy lover. He is a passionate, jealous God. His name is Jealous, it
says in Exodus 34:14. You need to stay out of the kitchen!

Who would want to trade back such a wonderful salvation? Who would want to be rescued from Egypt and go to the desert with God, a place where you learn to fall in love with Him, only to trade it back in for the wretched, threadbare, pathetic, and hopeless Egypt? In 1 Corinthians, the Apostle Paul cried out for us not to repeat Israel's history, saying, "These things happened to them as examples and were written down as warnings for us, on whom the fulfillment of the ages has come. So, if you think you are standing firm, be careful that you don't fall!" (1 Cor. 10:11–12).

Our hearts were programmed by God to love, to worship, to adore, to bow down. Remember, He has also saved us. He has saved us from having to love the food, and we get to love Him. He has given us an object for this affection that will not rob us or hurt us, but will promote us and benefit us. Half our battle is over because no one has to teach us how to love, how to worship, how to adore, how to bow down. The Israelites—God's children—are servants, slaves by birth. In fact, in the passage from Jeremiah we read earlier in this chapter, God says, "How *skilled* you are at pursuing love!" (Jer. 2:33, italics added). All we need to do is make a *choice* of what we adore. The plagues—especially the Passover plague, which is symbolic of the blood of Christ and the sacrifice of Jesus Christ, the Messiah, the Savior—have saved us from having to love this earth or anything on this earth or anything in heaven above—and we get to love God. Hallelujah! We get to love God! This is salvation!

He has given us an object for this affection that will not rob us or hurt us, but will promote us and benefit us.

So, repent because the kingdom of God is near. This means turn from your lover and turn toward God because God's heart is hovering over the face of the people. God's heart is near! It is near! We can reach His heart if we want it instead of trying to juggle two lovers. My friends, we may not always have this opportunity. Did God allow the wayward Israelites to return to Him? See for yourself. Let's go back to that passage in Jeremiah: "'If you will return, O Israel, return to me,' declares the LORD" (Jer. 4:1a).

Have you ever had anyone willing to fight for you? Well, I did one time, and it was great! I was at a prom, and I had broken up with my boyfriend and had accepted a date with one of his friends. Toward the end of the prom, my old boyfriend realized he really cared for me and wanted me back. In fact, he was even willing to fight for my hand. Well, it was resolved without any punches being thrown, but when it was all over, which one do you think my heart went out to? That's right—the one who cared for me and pursued my heart when he thought he might lose our relationship. He declared his feelings for me even though it might mean having to fight for what he cared about. Well, he was my hero at that time. That's how a hero is birthed in your heart. As I said earlier, God is a genius as well as the passionate pursuer of our hearts. He knows that men make heroes out of heavyweight champions, that mankind will follow the winning quarterbacks, that nations will throw confetti on the five-star general who strategically wins the battle, and that we will ride away anywhere with the knight in shining armor.

God is my Knight in shining armor, and God is your Knight in shining armor. No one has ever—and no one will ever—fight for the right of your hand in a covenant relationship as God Almighty has. He is the Hero we have all been dreaming of. He has fought for the right for our love and devotion, and since He has no needs, He has done it all purely for the glory of love! He has made you His precious choice. Why not make Him your choice and never backstroke the Red Sea again?

What You Can Do Today

- *Go where God is leading you in Scripture.*

- *Inspect your heart.* If you are feeling the pain of struggling, honestly examine your heart. Is this pain from true suffering due to dying to your will, or is it the pain of trying to keep hugging the refrigerator and asking God to repent? Is it the pain of sin?

- *Scrutinize your eating habits.* Each time you sit down to eat, ask yourself: Am I loving God and getting ready to enjoy His food, or am I getting ready to love and worship the food and only enjoy God? Begin focusing on God instead of the food.

- *Start over right now.* Do not wait until tomorrow morning or put it off until Monday. If you try to put it off, that means you really do not want to do it—in other words, you are making the choice to keep loving the food. Start over today by waiting until you feel physiological hunger (for instance, a stomach growl) before you feed the stomach again, and during that time of waiting for hunger, focus on God with all your heart and mind. Stay in God's Word.

- *Examine your focus.* You will fall in love with what you focus on. Make it easier to focus on God and Jesus Christ all day long. Learn the stories about God and Jesus that are in the Bible, notice the wonderful creation God has offered for us to live in, and seek out other people who are eager to discuss God and His will in their lives. Look for His guiding hand in your life today. It is there.

- *Make a list.* Count the ways God is your Hero so that you can fall in love with Him or so that He can become your very best Hero and Friend.

S'mores and a Way of Escape

In Weigh Down†, we believe that God provides a special "way of escape" when a person is tempted (1 Cor. 10:13). This way of escape was sent to us from a Weigh Down† participant:

Dear Weigh Down staff,

I started my camping vacation eating according to God's parameters of hunger and fullness. But I began to neglect my time in the Word, so it really didn't surprise me that I ended up "coasting" downhill with my eating. One day, my husband and daughter were taking a nap in the tent. I was reveling in my time alone, and instead of studying the Bible and praising God for His creation, I chose to read a novel and prepare a batch of s'mores: graham crackers with a melted chocolate bar and melted marshmallow—a campsite favorite! After all, no one was around to disturb my private indulgence. I started to eat my first s'more when I heard a loud hiss behind me. I turned around and was astonished to see a large black bear standing about three feet from me with his nose up in the air, looking very hungry! Well, I flung my s'more at him and dashed into our tent. "There is a bear out there!" I exclaimed. We watched the bear climb on top of our picnic table and eat the rest of the s'mores. In fact, he nearly licked the table clean! He even took the bag of marshmallows with him into the forest! At the time, my heart was pounding too fast to think this could be funny. But later, I was laughing, and I told my husband that God had gotten my attention with a really unique way of escape to get me back on track!

Sincerely,
Julie Pen—Portland, OR

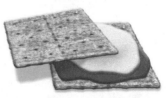

By the way, *I* would have been so terrified that I would never overeat again! Go, God!

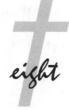

eight

HUNGER IN THE DESERT

*We must go through many hardships to enter the
kingdom of God.*

—Acts 14:22b

After God rescues you from the slavery of food, He takes you to the
Desert of Testing. Many people do well the first few weeks, but
when you realize God really expects you to eat less food, the heat of
the testing makes the desert seem impossible. You want out of this
hot test of self-denial. I hope that this chapter will give you the motivation for getting truly hungry—all the way to a growl.

> *Remember how the LORD your God led you all the way in the desert
> these forty years, to humble you and to test you in order to know what
> was in your heart, whether or not you would keep his commands. He
> humbled you, causing you to hunger and then feeding you with
> manna, which neither you nor your fathers had known, to teach you
> that man does not live on bread alone but on every word that comes
> from the mouth of the LORD.* (Deut. 8:2–3)

Without making a choice to go to the desert and allow yourself to
get truly hungry, you will never know God. Once firmly planted in

the desert, you're in the perfect environment to focus on God and know God and therefore love God. The desert is a place of passion and practicality. It's actually romantic because it is just you and God. But to get to know God, you have to get your focus on God and off Satan—and off the world.

There is another important ingredient once you are in the desert. As you just read: "God led you all the way in the desert these forty years. . . . He humbled you, causing you to hunger." You see, God *wants* you to get hungry. Now that God has taken you to the desert, He purposely wants you to get hungry, or to get empty. What does it mean to get hungry or empty?

When I first started teaching people about basic physiological hunger, it surprised me how few people had experienced emptiness. Emptiness is so fundamental. But I soon realized that to many, this was an unexplored concept. In The Weigh Down Workshop[t] seminar, I've spent several hours on video and audio, and in text, describing exactly what physiological hunger is. People will tell you that you will get sick if you wait for hunger. I have even had Christian organizations turn down Weigh Down Workshop[t] seminars because I tell people that God designed our bodies to wait for hunger. It doesn't take long to realize that the *forces that be* are very much against your finding, understanding, and experiencing this physiological hunger. Why is this so?

Emptiness is so fundamental. But I soon realized that to many, this was an unexplored concept.

As we have learned so far, Satan loves to confuse Egypt and the desert. But why would Satan want to cloud the concept of hunger, too? We must be on to something. This concept of hunger is very deep and encompasses much more than just physiological hunger. God said "to humble you and cause you to hunger." Humility means you are focused on God and expect nothing from anyone except Him. He wants humility hunger, which is intense, focused dependency. It also includes financial hunger, relational hunger, esteem hunger, directional hunger, and emotional hunger. The kind of hunger we are talking about is not merely a craving, a yearning, a hankering, or a want. In terms of food, it means bypassing your head hunger and desire eating and getting physiologically hungry—all the way to a growl. In terms of financial hunger, it may mean sometimes accepting beans and corn bread to eat. Manna for breakfast, manna for lunch, and manna for supper.

As we stay in the desert, this hunger evolves into a scarcity, a drought, a famine—in other words, a persistent need. It's a stripping down of the extras, down to the bare bone. About the time we think we can't lose anything else, there is something else to give up that we didn't even know we were attached to. This attachment reveals that we have loaded our security blankets with more than we ever dreamed—more than we thought a heart could hold on to.

Why Does God Want Us to Get Hungry?

Why would God want us to get hungry? Didn't He just rescue us from Egypt so that we can love Him in the desert? Yes, but we have been in Egypt a long time, dependent on the world and the world's remedies. God is going to have to deprogram us. There are pieces of Egypt stuck all over us, in between our toes and under our fingernails, and we are going to need a good scrub-down to wash this dependency upon the world out of our hair.

To Empty the Heart of Idols

During the Exodus, God told the Israelites to take articles of gold and silver and fine objects of value with them to the desert. They soon melted these items down and made them into a false idol. One of the reasons for this stripping under the new covenant is to prevent us from repeating history by taking the plunder of Egypt and melting it down into an idol—a golden calf. It is unthinkable to bring an idol to the desert of God, unthinkable to hang on to your food in the desert,

The principles of Weigh Down† are wonderful because they are so basic and so simple. I was immediately interested in the program since it seemed to complement many of the natural things we tell our patients to do postpartum and postoperatively. [I plan to] bring your program to other men and to my medical colleagues as well.

John Guarneri, M.D.
OB-Gyn
Winter Park, FL
Lost 31 lbs.

Obesity is considered an epidemic disease that 50 percent of the population has and there is no cure. There are programs that relieve symptoms for a short time, but they're not permanent. We will never find the answer in a medicine. We will never find the answer in a personal trainer or a wellness center that's going to train us three or four times a week. But Weigh Down† makes sense because it's the way God created us. You can get the desired medical benefits from eating this way.

Denise Sibley, M.D.
Internal Medicine
Johnson City, TN
Lost 70 lbs.

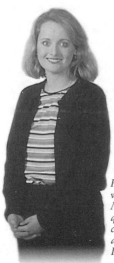

I like Gwen's direct approach in saying that you need to get right with God, and until you do, you just can't seem to move past your worship of food. I sincerely believe that through Weigh Down†, people who have never achieved or maintained weight loss will find success they never knew they could have.

Denise Williams, M.D.
Internal Medicine
Columbus, OH
Lost 16 lbs.

People need to realize that they can get by with a lot less food than they think they can. Many people do not realize that the consequences of overeating are often grave medical complications. Much of this could be avoided by obedience to God's eating plan. It really makes sense.

Tiffany Frazer, D.O.
Pediatrics
Miami, FL
Lost 33 lbs.

unthinkable to have to take crutches to make it through a desert day with just you and God. Just you and God should be *more* than enough. That relationship should be your everything, even though the world seems to be falling apart around you. How insulting to say, "God, You are putting me past what I can bear!" Some people turn to antidepressants for comfort, and that desire usually occurs when they are still in Egypt enslaved to the false god. Once you are truly in obedience to God in the desert, you drop your dependence on the world's remedies because you are so joyful to be under the enslavement of righteousness and out from under the enslavement of food.

To Know God as a Supplier

God wants us hungry to develop an alert focus on Him and a love only for Him. Hunger is a concept that unlocks and opens this door between you and God. Think about it. How could you ever know God if you don't get hungry? If you're always feeding yourself, how could you learn what it's like for God to feed you and learn how He feeds you and what He likes to feed you? How would you ever know that He loves blue cheese dressing, filet mignon, and sour cream on baked potatoes? How would you ever know that He loves Italian cream cake, chocolate cheesecake, and an ice-cream sundae with extra nuts? How would you know that He came up with all the different foods and created Fritos and dip for our enjoyment? Had you never gotten hungry in the program, eaten regular foods, and lost weight because of hunger, you would never know that God endorsed those foods. They would have remained evil in your eyes for the rest of your living days. This breakthrough was the result of getting hungry!

Likewise, if you never got all the way to lonely—by numbing this feeling with activity, antidepressants, or alcohol—you might never reach out and experience Him as an intimate companion. If you never had a financial need, you would never learn how miraculously He could provide. You would never know that He fixes roof leaks without anyone's help, and that He's a mechanic, He's a financier,

He's been known to pay rent, and He can mysteriously place ten dollars in your pocket. He's been known to calm creditors and heal or delay illnesses. I have found that He can find safety pins or car keys, He can coordinate outfits, and He is a great giver of good things. He has even answered my prayers to calm barking dogs in the middle of the night and to extend our food so that it is like the miracle of loaves and fish.

He is my resource for everything. I have gotten to know Him through many answered prayers. In fact, in the desert you find that He can creatively accomplish anything you can imagine to pray for in Jesus' name. There is something about the sweet name of Jesus— who has been entrusted with all authority because He is such a fan of God's. That is just like our God to give all authority to Jesus, and it is just like Jesus to tell everyone in John 14:31 that "the world must learn that I love the Father and that I do exactly what my Father has commanded me." I can look for a needed safety pin for five or ten minutes, but once I ask in the name of Jesus Christ, my eyes are opened, and there's the safety pin right in front of me. Is that not the nicest thing in the world?

Another natural result of getting hungry is the development of trust. Just think about it: when your babies cried, you fed them. When their diapers needed changing, you changed them. When their boo-boos needed a kiss, you kissed them. They had a need—you met their need. That's how they learned how to trust you and love you. And boy, did you ever fall in love with them while you were meeting their needs. You can't enter the kingdom unless you become like one of them.

You can't enter the kingdom without knowing God, and you can't know God without getting totally hungry and waiting for Him. If you're going to be your own god, you will never get to know *the* God. You'll do your own feeding, your own shopping, your own budgeting, and your own scheduling. How can you ever know God if you have never released your grasping hands, turning them palms up, and waiting for Him to fill them? If you never let go, how can you ever let God? Every day you do not wait for God to feed you, the less you will know about Him. The less you know Him, the less you love Him. The less you know about Him, the less you trust Him and the more inviting Egypt looks. If you would get hungry daily, you would find that love would grow, and *love* will keep you alive, not the food. Love between you and God will keep your heart beating. Egypt seems far away and food is not as interesting, but every word that comes out of the mouth of the Lord is cherished, and every move He makes is captivating.

To Examine if We Really Believe

Getting hungry is a concept that develops *belief.* Paul proclaimed, *"Believe* in the Lord Jesus, and you will be saved" (Acts 16:31a, italics added). Letting yourself get hungry really shows the heart. In other words, if you are having trouble getting hungry, it is because of a lack of belief that God has a good nature, that He has the best taste, and that He makes the best possible decisions. He's perfect. But when you are not so sure about that, it affects your behavior. If you don't get hungry and wait on His perfect timing for eating, Satan will always whisper, "God's not listening. He's in China. His watch is broken. He's forgotten you. God does not see you, and He is not here or there. God does not care." What happens next is that unbelief takes *root.*

If you would get hungry daily, you would find that love would grow, and love will keep you alive, not the food.

There are many lists of behaviors of unbelievers in the Bible. Let's look at Mark 7:21–23: "For from within, out of men's hearts, come evil thoughts, sexual immorality, theft, murder, adultery, greed, malice, deceit, lewdness, envy, slander, arrogance and folly. All these evils come from inside and make a man 'unclean.'"

Think about theft for a minute. Why would you ever steal or

cheat or lie about your time card at work if you believed in God? Why would you ever take a stapler from your desk at work? Don't you believe that God will get you one if you ask? We don't want to take the time to ask or to wait. If we did, why would we ever steal or cheat or lie? When we believe in God, we know about His desire to provide for those devoted to Him.

Most of us would not literally murder someone, but we might murder people with a look. Jesus said that if you hate someone, it is like murder. Why would you ever hate anybody if you believed in God? If someone did something against you, don't you know that God would make him miserable, and there is terrible judgment now and later? You don't have to hate if you believe in God. You are supposed to hate injustice or the sin—not the person. Your job description is to love God and to stay focused on Him. Watch how He pays back the people who do wrong. If you have waited for Him, you know: He's swift, He's decisive, and He's justifiably accurate when it comes to dealing with the wicked.

Why would you ever defend yourself if you believed that God could do a better job? If you believed in God, you would know He loves to defend you. Paul said in Romans 12:19, "Do not take revenge, my friends, but leave room for God's wrath, for it is written: 'It is mine to avenge; I will repay,' says the Lord." The act of taking revenge is not evil in and of itself, for God takes revenge. However, if *you* take it, you cannot watch God show off as He takes revenge on your behalf. You've missed a tremendous opportunity to watch our mighty Warrior woo you and court you by His heroism.

Nothing has made me trust Him more and fall more in love with Him than watching Him defend me from my enemies. David spent half the book of Psalms recounting God's sure defense. God allows enemies so that you can watch Him, like a passionate lover, fight for you. More than one-third of the psalms that David wrote are about David's crying out to God to defend him, or they are just beautiful demonstrations of how God was going to snuff out his enemies.

Look at Psalm 18:40: "You made my enemies turn their backs in flight, and I destroyed my foes." And Psalm 59:10b says, "God will go before me and will let me gloat over those who slander me." Or read Psalm 44:7: "You give us victory over our enemies, you put our adversaries to shame." Psalm 63:10 tells us that God will give our enemies over to the sword and they will become food for jackals. You see, King David knew the Father so well that he knew he would not have to take revenge because God does indeed defend the righteous. If you know God, you never have hate in your heart toward others because you know that when they do something wrong against you, God is going to punish them. Now, God may call you to have nothing more to do with them, and that is not wrong. After all, Titus 3:10 advises, "Warn a divisive person once, and then warn him a second time. After that, have nothing to do with him."

Here is another category: Why would we ever want someone else's spouse if we believed in God? Don't we believe that He can provide for our needs and wants? That is exactly why He was upset one time with King David. It was an insult for David to go out and get Bathsheba for himself. That was sin. Satan loved to laugh and say, "God, I don't believe You would give me more, and neither does Your servant King David. That's why he's sneaking behind Your back, and that's why I am. I don't like Your leadership."

There is nothing wrong with looking for a feeling. When you go to too much alcohol, it is a feeling you seek. When you go to too many cigarettes, it is a feeling. When you go to too much food, it is a feeling. When you look for too many material things, it is a feeling. Gossip—it is a feeling. Sexual lust outside marriage—it is a feeling. God programmed you to look for feelings, but only *He* can give you that feeling you are looking for.

Why would we ever be greedy for food or hoard money? Don't we know that God would give us food or more money if He wanted to? Why would we ever brag or show off? Don't we know that God is the One and only One who gives favor and takes it away? Why would we ever have malice or envy toward someone; why would we ever slander someone? If we believe in God, we don't have to promote ourselves, and we certainly don't have to tear someone down just to get where we want to go. Why would we ever have lewdness or immodesty if we believe promotion and favor come only from God? We don't know Him. Why would we ever lie if we know God would provide all things? We haven't experienced this, and we just don't believe in God's great personality and perfect leadership toward those who love Him. Unfortunately, we have been taught to fend for ourselves and to fight it out since birth.

Why would you ever have to control your spouse if you believe in God? When you believe in God, you know Him, and you know that all you have to do is let Him know what you want, and He will take care of it. You don't have to take care of it yourself or get your way. If people really knew God, why would they ever have any trouble submitting to their bosses? If women really knew God, why would they ever have trouble submitting to their husbands? If you stayed in the desert long enough and got hungry enough in your marriage relationship instead of jumping to divorce, you would know just how coordinated He is. He can fix anything and can fulfill everyone.

Here is an illustration that may help you learn to trust in God's balance of authority. A husband and his wife are sitting in the den at home. Everyone knows—especially marketers and advertisers—that men look at women and women look at women. God made it that way. That's why businesses use women for commercials to sell products. So, between the man and the woman sitting on the sofa, even though the man is in authority, the woman is going to get the attention. Her whims and wishes and opinions will be highly regarded. Children have much less authority than the woman and have to be submissive to their parents, but when a child walks into the room, all eyes are drawn to him or her. If there are several children, the attention goes to the youngest child, all the way down to the baby, who has the least authority of all and least wherewithal to defend or demand her way. (Actually, God has provided lungs that are highly capable of demanding attention when all else fails!) The child with the least ability to communicate seems to command the most attention. Even the smallest whimper will make everyone jump. But it doesn't stop there. Finally, a kitten wanders into the den. The kitten has no clout, a very low IQ, and no words. And yet all the attention in the room seems to go to the baby cat. And you'd better believe that the cat gets what it wants without even saying a word. So you see, God is the genius of balance and coordination, and when He tells us to submit, we have nothing in the world to be afraid of. This is one great God we serve who has thought of absolutely everything!

All of these behaviors we just discussed—evil thoughts, sexual immorality, theft, murder, adultery, greed, malice, deceit, lewdness, envy, slander, arrogance, and folly—are the behaviors of the unbeliever. Depression can result from a misguided focus on self or wanting more. Discontentment and emptiness arise in the unbeliever who doesn't know what a willing provider and generous giver God is. They don't know what a great protector and defender and fighter He is. They haven't noticed what a great rewarder and promoter He is. They don't believe, so they don't get. James 4:3 tells us, "When you ask, you do not receive, because you ask with wrong motives, that you may spend what you get on your pleasures," as opposed to using it to show how

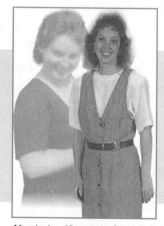

When I started Weigh Down†, we were in debt on credit cards because of greed. As I filled up my spiritual need with God's Word, I lost 48 pounds quickly. And after surrendering my will to God in spending money, we decided to cancel our credit cards and live by faith and use cash only. Within two weeks, my husband received a pay raise and bonus. We were able to pay off our debt, and now we have money in savings! God is our provider, and it's joyful to live in His excess.
Sarah Kojis—Elkhorn, WI

After losing 48 pounds, Sarah Kojis learned to entrust her finances to God.

great God is. They don't lay down their earthly love, and so they forfeit a relationship, the grace that could be theirs. The Bible teaches
us in Jonah 2:8 that "those who cling to worthless idols forfeit the
grace that could be theirs." They become greedy for their own food,
material possessions, and favor of man.

THE DILEMMA OF GREED

Some people cannot find a stomach *growl*—the truly empty, gnawing, burning sensation that feels so good, so right! I love to get to a
growl and then get what I really love to eat. How fun! Greed and
impatience are so juvenile and insulting to this incredibly good
Father of ours. How would you like it if your kids went around begging neighbors for bread or stealing something from their house,
explaining that they didn't believe you would give it to them if they
asked for it, or that you were too poor to give it to them, or that you
did not care enough about them to give them anything they wanted?
That would totally degrade your character as a loving parent who
wants to provide. So what have we done to God's character as a loving God? We have sinned, so God doesn't answer our prayers—but
we blame our Maker rather than change ourselves. Greed is indeed
idolatry. Peter denied his friendship with Christ three times because
he did not know God well enough or trust that God would defend
him and take care of him. However, God set Jesus on His right side
and made His enemies a footstool for His feet because Jesus believed
in God's great character and perfect leadership.

Incredibly, we invite people to church assemblies with us to meet
this loving God, but then we walk out the doors and we take revenge
when we are wronged because we don't believe God will defend us.
After church service, we run to excessive cigarettes, excessive alcohol, and continual antidepressants for comfort. We sneak extra food
at ten o'clock at night because we haven't experienced God filling us
up. We don't know Him! Then we nag our spouses if they don't do

what we want immediately, we sabotage our coworkers, and we try to control our family members. The nonbeliever we brought to church that day can see right through this. We just don't believe in a good God, and we haven't got a clue about how to tap into His resources. He owns the cattle on a thousand hills! Electricity everywhere—but we don't know how to plug into the Lord. Get connected! Fly that kite as Benjamin Franklin did, and tap into this invisible power that lights up and runs this world!

Fly that kite as Benjamin Franklin did, and tap into this invisible power that lights up and runs this world!

Someone who has meditated on and marveled at God's artistic hand, creative artwork, genius decisions, passionate heart, powerful strength, commanding presence, and His staff and resources *believes* in God. Young seekers who surrender their lives to the Father will begin to know about His system of justice. They learn to believe in Him as CEO of the universe. They develop trust that He is there for their own good, that He sees their needs, and that He is going to take care of them just as He has every animal, every bird, every fish of the sea, every baby, every child, every woman and man, every race—everyone.

When we don't know Him, we don't love or trust Him, and our lack of love makes us afraid that we are not going to be taken care of. But you can reverse this process. When you stay in the desert, you will learn to love and be loved, and perfect love casts out all fear (1 John 4:18a).

Having favor from God helps eradicate depression, and there is less anxiety since you have found the door to every resource. Depression and down feelings should be used to contemplate your path, to help you regroup or turn from a dead-end lifestyle of expectations from an idol—a false god. There is much diagnosed (and self-diagnosed) depression in this country. If you feel depressed—I warn you before you ever begin to consider this as one of the very rare chemical imbalances, such as an inborn error of metabolism or a genetic flaw—please consider God's world as a whole. If this depression is a chemical error, why does it show up so much more in America than in most other countries? Why do people in many countries who have fewer material things have more happiness, while the cost of depression in the United States is $43 billion a year?[1] Why isn't there widespread chemical imbalance in the animal kingdom? Why aren't more animals depressed? My dogs, Chaucer and Virginia, wag their tails every day. Every day! The birds sing their songs every day. I don't look out the window and see the cardinals still in bed with the shades down, feeling depressed. No! They chirp daily. Why is the most chemically impaired and more genetically flawed part of our population (people who are developmentally delayed) the happiest segment of our population? If anyone would have genetic or chemical imbalances, it would be them—but they are appreciative and happy as a whole. They haven't learned to be self-focused. We need desperately to change our attitudes, trust God, and stop worrying about chemical imbalances.

CONSISTENT HUNGER

How would you like to feel hunger day in and day out? How would it feel to never overeat again? Consistent hunger means you have developed consistent, trusting dependence on the Father, and getting to know God is everything. The deeper I delve into a subject, the more I see eternity. In other words, it removes the thought that heaven could ever be boring. God's creativity is endless. For example, take the universe. You can study the universe and the galaxies, but if you let your mind travel beyond the stars, it becomes hard to imagine. It speaks of infinity; it is unfathomable. It is so overwhelming that it could have two effects: (1) the beyond can make you feel afraid, or (2) the beyond can make you fall back into God's arms in faith. Some people look at the subject, but some people look at all things and see God. I believe that is how my faith has developed to the point that it has. I don't just hear a song; I hear a song and say to God, "I can't believe You are so poetic and Your music is so moving!" I don't just see a sky; I see a sky and tell God that I appreciate all the detail He went to today to make the sky so beautiful. I see God's handiwork, humor, genius, and judgment in everything. The invisible God has become very visible to me over the years.

In college, I studied what happens to peanut butter and jelly sandwiches after you eat them. I was awestruck when I studied all the different ways God had designed the intricate body systems that are self-sufficient, but that are sensitive to the other systems. More than 100 trillion cells are in the body, performing thousands of different roles and functions, all preprogrammed by God. Just think about it. When a baby is conceived, the cells begin to multiply from two cells, then separate into their own location and start functioning.

Let's look at *one* category of cells and their function: the antibodies. When an invading virus—whether it is one that causes the flu, smallpox, measles, or a cold—enters a body cell, it multiplies there. One virus can replicate itself 100 times in an hour. Those can then invade 100 other cells. Within hours, there can be as many as 10,000 virus particles invading 10,000 cells.[2] If this process is not stopped, it will overwhelm the body with disease.

Never fear! God has made our bodies to be able to detect a foreign cell. That's mind-boggling! I can't even detect when someone who doesn't belong is walking into our office, and I have eyes! The body recognizes this viral invader and manufactures a mirror image of the invader that attaches itself to the virus, thus rendering it ineffective. The first time this protein antibody is made, it takes several hours, so that you might feel the effects of the virus. This lock-and-key design is stored in molecular memory, so that the next time, your body will quickly recognize the same invader, manufacture the antibody, and attack immediately. This is known as immunity. In a normal, healthy individual, when a virus enters the body a second time,

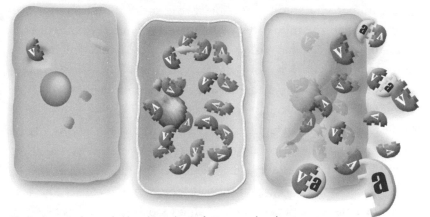

*The body recognizes a viral invader and manufactures a mirror image
of the invader that attaches itself to the virus, thus rendering it ineffective.*

the body responds rapidly since it has this antibody in its memory banks, and you do not even feel the virus's effects. You cannot be diseased by the same virus twice.

So are you amazed at how often you get sick? What should be amazing is how efficient and coordinated God's design of the body is—in other words, how often you *don't* get sick. It's almost as if every system has its own brain. I could comprehend this if we were attached by cords to the mainframe computer, God Himself, and our bodies were getting instructions through this umbilical cord. But we are all independent units, individuals walking around and able to reproduce another being.

What bothers me is the human tendency to study a subject and then worship the *created*—the intricacies of the human system—instead of the *Creator*. For instance, many of you might have just read this information and been amazed at the body rather than at the absolute, coordinated, genius ability of God. One perspective leads toward the fear I was talking about; the other perspective leads toward faith. Paul wrote about this in Romans 1:25: "They exchanged the truth of God for a lie, and worshiped and served created things rather than the Creator—who is forever praised."

The deeper you study any subject, the more complicated everything gets, and the more unexplainable it becomes. When you contemplate a subject and enter a door that goes way beyond your understanding, you have one of two reactions: you fall back into God's arms and trust in Him, or you fall back in fear.

One day, I was in a hurry to go to a speaking engagement, and at the last minute, my daughter Michelle told me that she needed a thermos. She gave me no ordinary thermos instructions; she asked that it be very large, and it had to have a drinking spout *and* a strap on it so she could carry it around at cheerleading camp. She also asked for a very particular type of shampoo. I needed a thank-you card for someone I would see that night, but I knew I didn't have time to get one because it takes me forever to pick those out. It was 3:13, and my speaking engagement was at 3:30. The stores would be closed by the time I got away from my speaking engagement, and to further complicate matters, Michelle's camp started the next morning. But I had to try.

On the way to a new drugstore that I was not familiar with, I prayed hard, and I prayed very sincerely: "God, I know that You made all the drugstores in the world, and God, I know that You have made all the products in the drugstores. God, I know that You have been the genius behind organizing every aisle and every product in this drugstore. I know that You know exactly where all of these products are. So, God, help me if You please." As soon as I got the prayer out of my mouth and stepped through the automatic entry doors, I was amazed that my eyes caught the sign for the shampoo at the very back of the store—at the very end of an aisle. And my eyes went right to this particular shampoo. Wow! I looked up and asked the pharmacist, "Where are your thermoses?" and she pointed to the aisle. And on the way to the thermoses were the greeting cards. The first card I opened—and this has never happened—was perfect. It said, "Thanks for the faith-lift," and I got it. When I got to the thermoses, my eyes went to the bottom shelf, and I saw a very large thermos with a drinking spout and a strap on it. There were eight people in the checkout line, but God reminded me of the sweet pharmacist in the back of the store who could check my items. At 3:31, I parked my car in the church parking lot. I believe in a coordinated, genius God and a sweet, caring, attentive Jesus. My respect for, belief in, and dependence upon God's skills and my willingness to go to Him for help were more than rewarded. I'm thrilled to know this God of ours. But I'm even more thrilled that the God of the universe would even one time in my life pay me any attention at all, much less listen to and answer my wishes that are not even matters of life and death.

WEIGHT LOSS WITHOUT TRUE HUNGER; RELATIONSHIPS WITHOUT TRUE LOVE

On the other hand, can we look as if we know Him, believe in Him and trust Him, and yet really not? Unfortunately, the answer is yes. In fact, you can lose one hundred pounds without ever getting hungry. You can imitate the behavior of a believer, but eventually, your true colors will shine through. Out of the abundance of the heart so the mouth speaks, and what is in your heart will surface. Can an employee work for you and never love you? Yes! Can a person walk out on his spouse after supposedly being "married" for thirty years with no explanation, no concern, and never call back? I've seen it happen. He had no love or foundation. As an employer of many employees, I've seen those who know me and believe that I look to the Father for guidance, and it may not always look as if what I'm doing is for the benefit of the employees. Those who stayed with me in the desert long enough learned that there were better times ahead. As an employer or as a parent, you cannot explain everything you are doing or every decision you have made.

I have learned that as time goes on, just about anything you do or say can be taken two ways, and Satan and his followers will use people to falsely accuse you. I have tasted just a piece of how God might feel, trying so hard to take care of and provide for and please people whom I love. Yet, in some instances, I've been misunderstood, misconstrued, falsely accused, and not loved back. No matter what I did, that friend, employee, or child wasn't happy. In some cases, you have experienced people who don't take the time to know you and would rather listen to Satan, who propagates the evil spirit of unbelief in God and His followers.

Can you be next to a loving person and not see him as loving? Satan was. Satan lived next to God in heaven, and he still didn't get to know God. It seems that Satan never wanted to understand the true character of God—a God who could show gentle love and passionate care while allowing suffering and hurricanes, division and judgment, wars and Hades. A lot of people don't even believe that God does send these things, but He *does*. Read the following passages: Isaiah 53:10a; Matthew 10:34; Amos 9:1–3; Isaiah 10:23; Ezekiel 6:6–7; Exodus 9:23–24; Zechariah 10:1a; and Jeremiah 30:23. These are just a very few of the many Scriptures in the Bible that talk about the awesome, destructive power of God.

I'm sure it was very painful for God to have to remove Satan from heaven. But Satan was misinterpreting everything and going around undermining God and planting seeds of doubt about God. The reason we've all had to experience this is that our dearest, most generous, and loving Father has had to live through centuries of people not wanting or seeing or trusting His loving nature.

His very being is love, yet Satan looked upon Him as the antithesis of love. Imagine that! Satan could not see what He was like. It is called *unbelief:* "To the pure, all things are pure, but to those who are corrupted and do not believe, nothing is pure" (Titus 1:15). Satan had to leave the heavenly kingdom, and he has been gathering a kingdom of hate around him that propagates this position of skepticism toward God and skepticism toward those who have a faithful allegiance to God.

When you consistently decide, *I'm going to eat,* but you're not at God's hunger point, you are your own boss. You've listened to Satan, and you've decided that you are your own god; you are your own provider. When you postpone your own control and relinquish decisions to God, you are in essence believing in God's timing, waiting for God's permission, blessing, and approval to go ahead. You are proclaiming silently to the world that you believe God and all His decisions are great! Sometimes, my children or my employees jump out ahead and do very good things, but they had not been given permission to go ahead. However, when a child or an employee receives permission, it makes her happy to have approval. This submission to authority makes everything work smoothly. Likewise, waiting for God's hunger and then eating what He puts in your heart and mind are foundational and increasingly beneficial.

They have discovered a great and profound mystery: submission to authority connects them with the one in authority.

Have you ever seen people who seemed perfectly content under submission—in fact, joyful and almost bubbling with life in that position? They have discovered a great and profound mystery: submission to authority connects them with the one in authority. The two now have a bridge to get to know one another, which results in becoming interwoven and united. Eventually, the employee, child, or one under authority will be blessed and promoted by the one in authority.

How many times has God cried out for you to just trust Him enough to allow this hunger experience and to open your mouth so that He can fill it (Ps. 81:10b)? How many times has He cried out for us to just get hungry and to give Him a chance so that He can take care of us and show us how adequate He is, how much He cares, and how much He is there for our own good? But Satan keeps crying, "Take care of yourself! No one else is going to do it!

Take care of yourself! You can do it! You can do a better job of feeding yourself!"

Well, we are cheating ourselves and wearing ourselves out, thinking that we can and should match the work of God. No, it's worse: we think we can do better than the work of God. We act as if we believe that *we* are gods. Again, how uninformed! Taking care of ourselves is the antithesis of believing in God. When we try to take care of ourselves, not only are we giving up the things we could learn— such as learning about God's character, learning to love Him, and learning to trust Him—we are also denying God the basic pleasure of feeding us and providing for us. If you have children, didn't you enjoy feeding your children? And yet we deny God this pleasure.

It's a Conviction Problem

You may have been in Weigh Down† classes for a while and know you need to get hungry, but you are just not waiting. You go to class and see others getting it; in fact, it seems that everyone *except you* is getting it. When you have obviously not lost the weight, you fool yourself by saying that Gwen said not to be "legalistic" about following hunger and fullness guidelines, but you are manipulating a truth so that you can indulge. When you are never hungry, that's not legalism; that's rebellion. You also say things like, "I must have a metabolism problem," or "My medical condition would not be benefited by hunger. In fact, it might make it worse." You tell yourself, "I have to eat with my family." You hear that freedom to eat whatever you want is "freedom," but you use it as a license to overindulge yourself with no boundaries. The end result is that you never experience consistent hunger.

You've tried to examine yourself. You may have gone back to the seminar workbooks and *The Weigh Down Diet*, thinking that maybe you missed something. You have talked to people who have "gotten it" in Weigh Down†, hoping that they could give you some new revelation. You felt yourself growing some spiritually, but not losing weight. You can tell faith is not all the way down in your heart, but for some reason, you stay in these small Bible studies, hoping they will stir you, but you never seem to change. What is wrong? It is called a conviction problem. You are not convicted that eating a few more bites is going to hurt God, or anyone for that matter, including yourself. *What does the Master of the universe care?* you think.

Well, being unconvicted, unconcerned, and overfed has been a problem for many. Some people are just "doubting Thomases." They are hardheaded and need everything in black and white and want to put their hands in the nail holes. I could tell you all day long that you are hurting God and that you are hurting yourself and your relationship with Him. But He needs to tell you. Ask God to show you.

One participant did just that. She asked God to make it clear to her—very clear. She wanted to know if overeating was indeed a sin. She thought she needed to see the word *sin* associated with overeating. She needed to see it in black and white. After praying for God to convict her, she opened her Bible (or let her Bible fall open) to the allegory in Ezekiel 16, where God referred to Israel as a baby girl whom He raised, loved, and clothed. But then she became a prostitute. The passage states, "Now this was the sin of your sister Sodom: She and her daughters were arrogant, overfed and unconcerned" (Ezek. 16:49). Well, there it was—the verse where "sin" and being "overfed" were linked. It moved the participant to repentance.

There are others who have told me of times they have felt overfed and unconcerned, so they cried out to God to scare them, so to speak, to put this "holy fear" back in their hearts. They knew they had become too casual with Him, and we cannot allow this to happen, for Isaiah 8:13a tells us, "The LORD Almighty is the one you are to regard as holy, he is the one you are to fear." God answered their prayers. Many times, the love stories I teach are not enough to move people to repentance. More than a few of God's people have been in the "fearless" state of mind. Look at this passage in Ezekiel:

As for you, son of man, your countrymen are talking together about you by the walls and at the doors of the houses, saying to each other, "Come and hear the message that has come from the LORD." My people come to you, as they usually do, and sit before you to listen to your words, but they do not put them into practice. With their mouths they express devotion, but their hearts are greedy for unjust gain. Indeed, to them you are nothing more than one who sings love songs with a beautiful voice and plays an instrument well, for they hear your words but do not put them into practice. (Ezek. 33:30–32)

Yes, we are unconcerned about overeating and unconcerned about getting truly hungry naturally. We manufacture hunger by taking pills. These pills are so brutal and damaging to the system that they make the system almost too sick to experience true physiological hunger. It is an artificial aversion to eating, not a heart that is submitting to God. True hunger is a wonderful experience, but we continually try to buffer it by feeding ourselves before we get physically hungry or by taking diet pills. We call our in-laws to help us if we are nearing financial hunger, take antidepressants when we become emotionally hungry, or numb ourselves altogether with excessive pills or alcohol. We are postponing knowing God, and therefore, postponing loving and trusting Him more.

God knows that desert hunger is a very fragile operation because once the vessel is stripped and the bone becomes exposed, the heart becomes extremely needy. That's the point: you *need* to experience *need*. However, Satan realizes this God-driven desert operation is a susceptible time, and he will rush in to offer you anything and everything on the earth to fill up this void because the world is his to offer. Satan will say, "It's too hot in the desert—make it easy on yourself and don't go all the way to hunger. Mix this hunger with some of *your* decisions. Get on that man-made diet and try waiting for hunger *some* of the time. Waiting for the hunger signal is too much of a time-consuming battle. Instead, just diet, eat certain foods, avoid other foods, and increase your exercise . . . and take some pills, too."

Jesus was totally focused and in love with God in the desert, so He was able to quickly turn down the phony pacifiers that Satan pushed. It was repulsive for Him to put food or power or material things into His heart, for His heart was full of love for God.

MANNA FROM THE FATHER

God humbles us, causing us to hunger, and then, He feeds us with manna. We must be willing to receive God's love once we are in the desert. This relationship, or this manna, will fill the void. This love runs your very life. No longer save yourself. No longer feed yourself. No longer save yourself from the hunger with pills. Let Him save you.

It was repulsive for Jesus to put food or power or material things into His heart, for His heart was full of love for God.

God has put me through severe testing and struggles in the dry, thirsty desert with many things. I was tempted to help myself, but God showed me that it was His will that I did not save myself or help myself. I clung to the stories of Job and of Jesus. But in my darkest hour, God's approval was what drove me, but faith that things would get better is what got me through. Accepting suffering is a must.

When Jesus was in His darkest hour on the cross, with the nails in His hands and feet, the people tempted Him to save Himself. Luke 23 tells us that

> the people stood watching, and the rulers even sneered at him. They said, "He saved others; let him save himself if he is the Christ of God, the Chosen One." The soldiers also came up and mocked him. They offered him wine vinegar and said, "If you are the king of the Jews, save yourself." . . . One of the criminals who hung there hurled

insults at him: "Aren't you the Christ? Save yourself and us!" (vv. 35–37, 39)

"Take care of yourself! Stop putting yourself down! Change how you think about your overeating and yourself!" These are all the cries of the false prophets. This advice will let you stay just as you are. But if you truly love yourself, not peace or popularity, but just you and your soul, you will move yourself right back into the hot (but incredible), submissive relationship with the only good God in the world. What is God's interest in man that He tests us so? Or as Job 7:17–18 puts it, "What is man that you make so much of him, that you give him so much attention, that you examine him every morning and test him every moment?" For the answer, consider Jesus.

Jesus, unlike us, had all authority but believed in God's perfect decisions so much that He would not consider the option of saving Himself from His terrible predicament. Again, saving yourself screams to the world that you don't believe in a God, especially the good God. Jesus' dying on the cross proclaimed to the world that He believed in an incredible and glorious Father.

God wants us to believe in Him. There is only one way to find Him, and that is leaving Egypt behind and following Him to the desolate desert in a surrendered position. There is only one way to love Him, and that's to get to know Him. There is only one way to get to know Him, and that's by truly getting hungry. Getting hungry starts this cycle of growth, and this cycle gives Him a chance to show off. You can now see how He looks, how He moves, how He thinks, how He responds, how He listens, and how He loves. You know Him and you like what you see, and your heart starts to pound harder for Him. It is the result of the desert journey.

So if God wants this for us, if He wants hunger, then we should want it, too! How do we get hungry? Good question. It's one thing to allow ourselves to get hungry one time. But it's another to stay in the desert and allow ourselves to get hungry daily. As it says in Isaiah

58:5a: "Is this the kind of fast I have chosen, only a day for a man to humble himself?" No—God is asking for us to stay humble and to stay dependent on Him, and a way to show this is to allow ourselves to

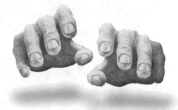

get hungry every day. It is best described by taking grabbing hands and turning them palms up all your living days. Take greedy hands off the food, money, and anything in this world.

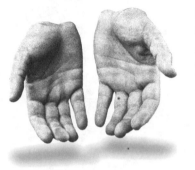

Those who make it through the dry, thirsty land will find a relationship that they will not trade for gold or silver or life itself. Even though God describes the journey as a "vast and dreadful desert that is thirsty and waterless," the thirst is quenched with a relationship and the hunger is filled with love. The more you have to surrender in the desert, the more you will fall in love with God. I almost lose my breath when I think He is trying to get my attention now.

There was once a Man who would sit on the side of a hill and tell stories so that you could find out what the heavenly Father was like, so that you could know Him and learn to fall in love with Him, too. The stories were powerful stories about things such as how the Father loves the prodigal son and how He is attentive to His sheep like a shepherd. Once He sat down on a mountainside and began to preach:

> *Blessed are the poor in spirit,*
> *   for theirs is the kingdom of heaven.*
> *Blessed are those who mourn,*
> *   for they will be comforted. . . .*

Blessed are those who hunger and thirst for righteousness,
for they will be filled. (Matt. 5:3–4, 6)

Trust Jesus and make a vow to get hungry, for when you get all the way to hungry, you will find that all you need is His love, and that love relationship will keep you alive!

What You Can Do Today

- *Go where God is leading you in Scripture.*

- *Wait for hunger.* God intends for us to feel physiological hunger. It is the way our bodies are designed to work, but more important, it is the way we can come to trust that God will provide for us. Today, make it a point to let yourself get truly hungry. You will love the way you feel!

- *Count your blessings.* Think about all the "hungers" God has had you experience in the past (physical, financial, emotional, etc.). Make a list of the awesome things God has done for you in your times of deepest hunger and need. As you look over your list, take some time to pray and thank God for being such a wonderful and attentive provider.

- *Help those around you.* If you are feeling depressed, try this experiment: go one full day—from the time you open your eyes in the morning until your head hits the pillow at night—focusing on taking care of the needs of others and asking God for His guidance in this area. Be determined not to focus on yourself. At the end of the day, you will feel refreshed, revitalized, and renewed!

- *Find true fulfillment.* There is nothing wrong with searching for a feeling, but overindulgence in food or anything else on this earth is *not* going to fill you up. What are some of the ways that you feel (physically and emotionally) after you overeat or binge? None of these feelings are the true feeling you were searching for in the first place. Look to God instead, for only He can fill your seeking heart!

_____

_____

_____

Home for the Holidays

There's nothing like getting together with family and special friends, especially at Thanksgiving and Christmas. All the bakeries display a festive array of cakes, pies, cookies, breads, and other tantalizing treats. And who can resist the smell of fresh bread baking, turkey roasting, or glazed ham baking in the oven? These special occasions also tend to revive old family recipes from past generations that can sometimes tempt us to binge. One tip to help you rise above the binge is to first survey all the food and know what is available. Then you can choose the foods that will be the most appealing to you at mealtime. After you have surveyed the food, you can select your favorites—a piece of glazed ham instead of turkey and dressing, and sweet potatoes with marshmallows instead of the mashed potatoes and gravy. You add some green beans and a dinner roll, and decide to wait on dessert for now. Now you are ready to enjoy your holiday meal. Since you have already surveyed the food and selected your favorites, you can now rate the selections on your plate. Remember to eat the best bites first; you *don't* have to clean your plate! When you feel yourself approaching fullness, push the plate aside or simply cover it with your napkin. Remember to save room for your favorite dessert later. What if you are not hungry when the holiday meal is served? Just fix your plate, cover it, and set it aside for later. You'll enjoy it much more when you are truly hungry. And here is another tip: *ask* for your favorite recipes! Most of the time, the person who prepared the dish is honored and will be very happy to share the recipe. Then you can prepare those family favorites and enjoy them *any* time of the year, not just at the holidays.

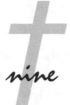

nine

SAVE YOUR HEART FOR ME

When I was a little girl and falling in love with God, I would think about Him and talk to Him all the time. He has always been very real to me, and I have always wanted to be close to Him.

YOU ACT A LITTLE SILLY WHEN YOU FALL IN LOVE

One thing I loved to do as a little girl was to imagine that heaven was a big square pasture. I would say, "God, if You'll just let me into heaven, I'll stay way back in the far pasture, and that would be fine with me. I would be so happy, God!" Well, I grew older and got to know Him better, and the next thing you know, I was trying to inch toward His castle. I was actually imagining myself getting closer to God. I told God, "Please, if You will just let me into Your castle, I'll do anything. I'll even clean the bathrooms." I was willing to do anything to be a little closer to this magnificent King. I loved Him so much, being far away wasn't going to work. As I have continued to fall more and more in love with Him over the years, I have continued to ask God if I can get closer to Him.

My love for God fills my heart, and one of the things that I have always done is sing songs to God. There is one song in particular that I have been singing to Him for about twenty years. Whenever I hear certain songs, whether they are country, pop, or Christian, I know that God is singing them to me, and I echo in response to His love songs. When I was a child and imagined inching toward God's castle, there were times that I would worry that since God loved everybody, there might not be a room left for me in the castle. I wanted to make sure He saved a place for me. So, this is a short little song that I would sing to God:

> *Walk along the lake, with someone new.*
> *Have Yourself a summer fling or two.*
> *But remember I'm in love with You,*
> *So save Your heart for me.*
> *When the summer moon is on the rise,*
> *And You're dancin' under starlit skies*
> *Please don't let the stars get in Your eyes,*
> *Just save Your heart for me.*
> *When You're all alone, far away from home,*
> *Someone's gonna flirt with You*
> *I won't think it's wrong if You play along,*
> *Just don't fall for someone new.*
> *When the autumn winds begin to blow*
> *And the summertime is on the go*
> *You'll be in my arms again I know,*
> *So save Your heart for me*
> *Father, save Your heart for me.*[1]

Even as a child growing up in the world, I have done some crazy-sounding things because of my love for God. You have already read about my early beginnings when I developed the Weigh Down† program, and I would tell people to "chew on this" while handing them a Bible. At first, people seeking my help would laugh at this bit of advice, but at least they *would* try what I was suggesting. The results were amazing.

Many would come back weeping as they experienced initial communications with the God of the universe. They had plugged into something incredible when they *turned from* food and *turned toward* God. God responded. This is *deep*—very deep. See, when you leave your lover behind, God will communicate with you. But if you choose another lover again, you will find the communication diminishing. Most people do not ask other people to chew on the Bible, but God was blessing my unorthodox approach.

LEARNING TO LOVE AUTHORITY

God has led me through many experiences since those early days that have helped me to learn about the heart of man and the heart of God. I had already experienced being a child *under* authority of parents, a wife *under* the authority of a husband, an employee *under* the authority of employers, and a student *under* the authority of teachers—and as those of you who have pursued higher education know, you sometimes have to submit to some pretty strange characters. On the other hand, I had also experienced being a mother who had authority *over* her children and being an instructor who had authority *over* college students. With Weigh Down†, God gave me a new experience *over* coordinators of classes and authority *over* adults at work. There have been great times, but there have also been some trying times because I was so green and inexperienced.

You may have also been put into positions of responsibility for making decisions, trusting people, and providing for people, so you already know what I am talking about. Looking back on it, I know now that God wants all of us to experience being in authority so that we can know exactly how He feels. Anyone who has been in a supervisory position over many people has the utmost respect and sympathy for God as a leader who has to make tough decisions. My heart goes out to God, and there have been several times that I have wept with Him over how painful it must be to supervise this wild group of people who have varying levels of devotion down here on earth.

The main thing I have learned is that as an employer, I automatically love anyone who says she wants to come to work for me. I mean, I can hardly get my kids to make their beds, so as this fresh, new employer, it made my heart sing to think that anyone would want to help me in any way. It just so happens that I have had mostly incredible, positive experiences with my employees because so many of them went through Weigh Down† first, and they have already identified their stronghold and understand dying to their will. But we all know that there are many painful and awkward relationships that ultimately expose the heart of man.

I have been on the other end of the line of authority most of my life—that is, I've been an employee most of my life. And if an employee has it together, she understands who is paying her salary, who is providing the benefits, and who is able to fire her. If Christians understand their position correctly, they understand who makes their hearts beat, who provides their very source of life, and who has the authority to unplug that source. God didn't put us on earth to learn to be good employees. There will be no Wall Street corporations in heaven. Small business owners will not be taking their businesses with them to the next life. God wants us to understand why He is in authority and to become accustomed to lines of authority. He is testing us to see if we can recognize His genius behind this setup and to see if we can joyfully get with the program. Truly submitting means that you are a team player, you think the Coach is great, and even if the assignment seems unusual, you obey it. When the Israelites reached the Promised Land, they were so confident of God's unique and competent leadership that they did not flinch when God told them to walk seven times around a city and blow a horn for the fall of Jericho. These desert survivors were definitely Promised Land material. The evidence is in their focus: they had to be focused on God. If they had the slightest focus on themselves, they would have been merely people walking in circles blowing on a horn, but instead they witnessed the wall of Jericho crumble by the mighty hand of God.

Whenever you unplug yourself from God's line of authority, you experience the threshold of confusion and the absence of peace. God gives us parent-child relationships not just so we can have a lot of children, but so we can learn who He is and how He feels toward us, how crazy He is about us, and how much pain He goes through if we insist on the path of the prodigal son. Some children have to come unplugged to understand how great it is to be plugged in. It is how we learn about God.

God wants us to understand why He is in authority and to become accustomed to lines of authority.

Likewise, God gives us the husband-wife experience so that we can once again know how passionate He is for us, and it helps to explain our covenant relationship with Him. The marriage experience can be the best university or schooling of all, and it lets us learn to focus on the few characteristics that are essential to maintain that relationship with Him. God didn't put males and females on earth to be good at being a man or a woman. The Bible indicates there won't be either male or female in heaven—just hearts in love with God. God didn't put marriage on earth just so we can get good at marriage! Marriage is not an end in and of itself. First of all, Jesus did not even get married, and He said there would be no marriages in heaven. In Matthew 22:30, Jesus declared, "At the resurrection people will neither marry nor be given in marriage; they will be like the angels in heaven." Marriage is one of the most vivid pictures of our relationship with God, this agreed-upon relationship we have with Him. It is as strong as the father-child relationship. Every thing and every experience is a shadow of what is to come. And since the best teacher is experience, God has devised all these adventures from birth to death so that we can know who He is. He is the King; He is not going to change. We need to get that straight if we are seeking to be in His kingdom. All other selfish goals and ambitions fall by the wayside as we learn everything it takes to maintain a good marriage or covenant relationship.

The Mysterious Link Between Authority and Devotion

God gives parent-child, husband-wife, employer-employee, and teacher-student relationships to expose and dispose of any undevoted or disloyal characteristics that might surface. Vertical devotion is the key—all the way up the ladder to God Himself. Are you devoted to the ones God has given you on earth to be devoted to? Are you devoted to anyone besides yourself and your stomach? Does your spouse or your parents or your employer say that you are a devoted or loyal person?

Through my experience, I have seen wholeheartedly devoted hearts. I have also seen semi-devoted hearts, selfish hearts, two-faced hearts, deceitful hearts, wishy-washy hearts, clogged hearts, and secretly ambitious hearts. When I see all the possibilities for defective hearts, I don't blame God for making an earth to put us on to help us work through a lot of these abnormalities before we are in His presence or His tearless heaven. I personally don't blame Him for staying invisible during this process of elimination!

Everyone—if you have lived any time at all—has experienced some level of the hurt or pain that God feels from rejection. Think about it from God's perspective. Can you imagine getting shown up by a bowl of cheese dip and chips? I can't even comprehend how He has been able to put up with all of the grief we've given Him, for it is the person who loves the most who will feel the most pain. It's the parent who has birthed and poured out her life for that wayward child who suffers the most. It's the spouse who has tried everything he knows to make his mate happy, and yet the mate still walks out on him, who grieves the most. It is the boss who automatically loves anyone willing to work for him who is tormented the most if someone turns out to be undedicated.

Horizontal vs. Vertical Devotion = Disaster

In almost all the cases of defective hearts or disloyal hearts, the common denominator is going to be that the undevoted person's heart has wandered to a horizontal—versus vertical—devotion. Oh, it looks religious and godly, but it is actually lethal to all relationships. "Horizontal" is a focus on what man thinks, and "vertical" is a devotion to what God thinks. A child who has moved to a horizontal devotion cares more about what his peers think than what his parents think. Eventually, it permeates every decision he makes, from clothing selections to choices of friendships.

In the same way, spouses can be cruel. I see many couples make a lifelong, devoted commitment to one another, then daily make the decision to side with the children at the expense of the spouse's feelings. Sometimes they allow their hearts to wander to coworkers at their jobs. They've moved from a vertical to a horizontal devotion, and it wreaks havoc. I've seen employees become more devoted to one another than to the employer, to the point of teaming up against the manager. It's horizontal versus vertical.

To me, it is a cancer that permeates Americans. The understanding of the line of authority has become so far removed from our basic character that it almost seems it is wrong to be under authority. Nowadays, the person in authority is automatically suspect and is not to be trusted. However, God wants us to make correct judgments and then submit to leaders that He has authorized.

It is common practice to chronically scrutinize, examine, and judge the ones in authority. After all, hasn't Hollywood consistently implied in movie after movie that employees are more moral and smarter than the owner of a big business, and that all women are more capable than all men, and that all children inherently have more sense and morals than all adults—especially parents—and that animals are smarter than people altogether, and finally, that wisdom lies in nature—in other words, that trees and stars house truth? We have bought into Satan's ploy to automatically undermine all authority to the point that we're not so sure that God designed and placed all authority and all people in leadership, even the pharaohs in the world. God is the One who lifts people up, and He is the One who sets them down (Dan. 2:21a). The Bible states, "Everyone must submit himself to the governing authorities, for there is no authority except that which God has established" (Rom. 13:1a).

Children obeying their parents are practicing obeying God. Women submitting to their husbands are, in essence, submitting to God. Men who submit to authority at work are showing that they believe in God. Ephesians 6:6–7 says, "Obey them not only to win their favor when their eye is on you, but like slaves of Christ, doing the will of God from your heart. Serve wholeheartedly, as if you were serving the Lord, not men."

We do not know who is paying the salary anymore, who is footing the bill, who is backing the life-support system, who is bringing home the bacon, or in some cases, who is cooking the meal. Do we just think an endless supply of backers, sponsors, or benefactors is out there? What's wrong with us? Do we think we can just walk out and obtain another set of parents, another husband, another wife, another employer—another God? First John 4:20 says, "If anyone says, 'I love God,' yet hates his brother, he is a liar. For anyone who does not love his brother, whom he has seen, cannot love God, whom he has not seen." Likewise, if you can't submit to your boss, whom you do see, you can't submit to God, whom you don't see. God is in authority.

You may think, *Well, that's not me. I mean, I don't really care for my boss, and I'm not really going to do what my husband says to do, and my parents are so out of it that anyone could understand why I limit my time with them. But I'm not being antiauthority.* You excuse yourself as being a partially devoted spouse or a marginal employee, but I'm here to tell you that there is no "partially devoted" category or "marginal" category. There's no such thing as divided devotion, for either you will love the one and hate the other, or you will be devoted to the one and despise the other.

This has such deep implications for explaining a Promised Land. It is *impossible* for you to serve *both* God and food. What wonderful news: as you love God, you will not be able to bow down to the brownies! It will be repulsive to eat the second half of the hamburger. You will despise worshiping the food. You *cannot* serve both God and someone or something else; therefore, the Promised Land is in sight—you will lose weight!

I've had employees tell me that they feel frustrated working for a particular supervisor, but they don't know where their uneasiness is coming from. They feel some resentment, and they even express anger at doing the task at hand. Nine times out of ten, it boils down to the fact that the employee has become more devoted to something or someone else—or just devoted to self—not the supervisor to whom she should be devoted. So they automatically hate and disdain the one they are not devoted to: the one in authority. It causes a source of strain. It pulls them away from who they are really devoted to—King Self. It is horizontal versus vertical devotion. People are afraid not to serve self, but I am here to tell you that I have cast everything I have out to the world to try to help others, and it has come back to me a hundredfold.

Antiauthority Develops Fear and Eventually Hate

In years of counseling people about their weight, many issues have come up, including marriage concerns. I have had people tell me that they just can't figure out why their spouse frustrates them so or where their feelings of hate are coming from. As I delved deeper, I learned that they were not devoted to their spouse, but they were

Before Weigh Down†, I believed that it was my fate to be fat, over 300 pounds! However, from the beginning, the truth about my condition was made clear to me, and this message about being set free from loving the food spoke to my heart. Losing the weight has been a natural side effect of my growing relationship with the Lord. I am so grateful to know Him better.

Deborah Prescott—Minot, ME
Lost 170 lbs.

My prayer every day is for my focus to be completely on obedience to God in every area of my life, especially to hunger and fullness. It is how He designed me, and I desire to be obedient to Him. Some say, "You can lose the weight, but can you keep it off?" My answer is, "Absolutely!" God has removed the stronghold and the fear. The weight is lost forever. Praise God!

Sherri Lomas—Anacortes, WA
Lost 128 lbs.

I weighed almost 300 pounds, and I was done trying to lose weight through diets when my wife introduced me to Weigh Down†. The Lord drew us both into this desert journey of dying to our self-will. He showed me that I was worshiping food and it was an idol in my life. I realized that the weight wasn't the issue, but that it was always an issue of the heart, and there was a strong bondage there. As God took me through the process of dying to the flesh, there was always freedom on the other side.

Ron & Amy Kalebaugh
Eldena, IL
Ron lost 100 lbs.
Amy lost 38 lbs.

devoted to the man or the woman at work or to the sport they adored. Again, they were simply devoted to themselves.

It's the same with food. If you are still fighting the battle and struggling with losing weight, your conflict and anger come from trying to obey God when your heart is still obeying the food. It is an automatic response or normal behavior of the heart of mankind.

There is nothing wrong with *hate* in and of itself. Many Scripture references point out how the righteous hate dishonest gain, and even God Himself points out that He hates sin. God Himself said, "I have loved Jacob, but Esau I have hated" (Mal. 1:2b–3a). So the emotion of hate or despising is not wrong. We are to be devoted to God first, and then God makes our hearts automatically hate the other lovers. Submission to the line of authority is the sure way to show your devotion to God. Likewise, horizontal commitment is the sure way to show that you despise God. It is the fail-safe way to express your rejection of God Almighty.

You might complain, "Gwen just does not understand my situation. My spouse is not a Christian. My employer is unethical. My life is so stressed," or "I have been so abused that I am justifiably devoted to food versus God." Well, you don't know the Father. He allows difficulties. You don't learn submission to your will under a like-minded person in authority. Your heart is not tested in the desert under optimum circumstances. This is exactly a part of the genius plan of God. He is going to allow your heart to be tested by fire. But it doesn't last too long if you choose vertical devotion over horizontal devotion at every test.

Let's look at this familiar passage in Exodus 20 more closely. God says:

I am the LORD your God, who brought you out of Egypt, out of the land of slavery. You shall have no other gods before me. You shall not make for yourself an idol in the form of anything in heaven above or on the earth beneath or in the waters below. You shall not bow down

to them or worship them; for I, the LORD your God, am a jealous God,
punishing the children for the sin of the fathers to the third and fourth
generation of those who hate me, but showing love to a thousand gen-
erations of those who love me and keep my commandments. (vv. 2–6)

So we will be either in the category of those who hate God or in
the category of those who love God. There is no middle ground. If
you love the food, you will automatically despise suggestions for eating less food, much like the undevoted employee who despises his
supervisor. You will find the task at hand hard to do, and you will
keep seeking other people to explain to you how to eat less food. For
example, you will continually ask, "What is hunger?" and "I'm still
not sure where full is." You will claim you cannot understand the
message because you have a hard time understanding my southern
accent. You will ask questions like, "What does Gwen really mean by
'empty'?" or "What does she mean by 'being submissive to your husband' or 'dying to your will'?" Since you love food and reject or
despise God, you cannot comprehend how to serve Him.

How to Make Letting Go of Food Easy

It is *easy,* not work, to serve the one you love. If your husband loves
golf, does he say, "What does it mean to use a nine iron? Well, why
do I have to practice putting?" No! It is a delight! If you love golf, it
is a delight to talk about it, plan for it, shop for it, and practice it. The
person who loves food rapidly catches on to counting every fat gram,
studying the food list, shopping for the food, preparing the food,
cooking the food, and consuming the food because it is the object of
affection. It is easy to serve the one you love, but it will always be a
problem to understand how to serve the master you despise or reject,
or who comes in second place. It will always be impossible to stop
serving the one you truly love. It will always be impossible to joyfully and competently serve the master you despise.

That is the behavior of love. You can't work your way to heaven. If you love God, you will willingly obey Him. It won't be work or a chore. Stop working on the "have-to" obedience, and start working on the foundation of whole love. The obedience will follow. Fix the direction of the heart, and your body will lose the weight! Once you have made the choice—that's the big thing—obedience will help you love. In 1 John 2:3–6, the Bible says, "We know that we have come to know him if we obey his commands. The man who says, 'I know him,' but does not do what he commands is a liar, and the truth is not in him. But if anyone obeys his word, God's love is truly made complete in him. This is how we know we are in him: Whoever claims to live in him must walk as Jesus did." Study this passage and you will see obedience feeding love, and love feeding obedience. God is the key to freedom and life, and you must never change this choice of master. You can't jump from making food your master to making God your Master, then jump to King Self, then back to the food god, and then back to *the* God without massive confusion and depression. Remember, Cain tried this and was angry and depressed.

It will always be impossible to stop serving the one you truly love. It will always be impossible to joyfully and competently serve the master you despise.

Oh, the joy of the ones who choose God and therefore obey their parents, submit to their spouses, and wholeheartedly honor their employers! They will experience the fact that parents can't wait to shower their children with blessings. It's a good thing children can't ask for the car keys when they are babies because a parent would try to accomplish even that request. You don't have to tell parents to love; they just do. Generally, you don't have to tell husbands to love their wives—husbands love to please their devoted sweethearts. (Now, I'm sure there are exceptions!) And usually, employers want their employees to be happy and well taken care of. And in turn, they would like the employees to love them back. You don't have to worry whether God loves you—He can't help it.

THE STORY OF CHAUCER AND VIRGINIA

I have two dogs, Chaucer and Virginia, and I have learned a lot of lessons about God and His will through these puppies. I have never seen loyalty like a dog's to its master. They have eyes for only one master. They know your voice, and they will sleep as close to you as you will let them. With my dogs, just saying, "Back, Virginia! Back, Chaucer!" will not keep them from slobbering all over me. I almost have to push them away because they adore me so much.

After our family moved to Nashville, we had to live in a little guest house while we were renovating the main house. This little guest house was near our next-door neighbor's horse stable, and the girls at the horse stable really wanted our collies to come over and play with them. I let them call the dogs across the fence, but I warned them never to feed the dogs. I was so busy with overseeing the renovations, building a new office building at Weigh Down†, writing *The Weigh Down Diet,* and going on the book tour that by the time I came home from the book tour I had no dogs. At first, I could call them and call them. Finally, they would come over for a few minutes, but as soon as I turned my back, they ran back to the barn. Of course, I wonder why—the stable just had girls—and horses—and I'm sure there were leftover lunches and all kinds of dog treats! My dogs were in Egypt!

My dogs had chosen a new master. So how was I going to compete with Egypt? I could hardly get them to stay home long enough to know how much I loved them and how badly I wanted to take care of them and feed them wonderful scraps from the table. I would call them, but eventually, my voice was nothing more than the wind blowing to my dogs. I couldn't get the dogs to come at the sound of my pleading at all. I was heartbroken. Every day, when I drove up my driveway from work, I longed to see my dogs greeting me as they used to, but they were gone!

I tried to get the girls at the barn to stop being so affectionate to the dogs, but the fact was, most of them already had. Chaucer was no longer a puppy, and he wasn't the cute little thing that he had been. In fact, he was chewing up their riding habits. But the girls were busy and unconcerned. Know this: you cannot count on Egypt to kick you out. You can't count on the very thing that has seduced you to lead you out again. And rest assured that the magnet that lured you into a relationship is probably no longer even there. The enticement is gone, but now you are trapped.

> You cannot count on Egypt to kick you out. You can't count on the very thing that has seduced you to lead you out again. And rest assured that the magnet that lured you into a relationship is probably no longer even there. The enticement is gone, but now you are trapped.

Virginia was older and more established in her devotion to us, but Chaucer did not know who his master was. And it was even more involved than I thought. After daily trips to the fence line to call Chaucer home, I noticed a horse trainer at the barn. I would see her with Chaucer every day, and I noticed Chaucer following her around all day long. Finally, I caught up with her and told her that Chaucer was not her dog and to please send him home. I even encouraged her to take a newspaper and bop him on the tail end. She said that she "would never do something like that," implying that I was a dog beater and an inadequate master. She obviously wanted Chaucer and indicated to me that she couldn't do anything about it because Chaucer had made his choice. He was sitting by her side as we spoke, and she was petting his head. I was embarrassed to death because I couldn't even get my own dog to come to me. Chaucer followed her back into the stable. I was jealous, and a silent war was declared that day. I wanted my dog home, and I wanted a chance to prove that I was the loving master. But I must admit, I was insecure about my getting a chance to do so.

Well, it took weeks of doling out special treats, leashing the dogs, loving the dogs, releasing the dogs, going back to the barn to get the dogs, fussing at the dogs, and starting all over again. Eventually, the memory of Egypt faded, and the lure of the girls and the horses is almost history. There were many times that I couldn't spot Chaucer immediately when I came home from work. I would run out and search for him, and be delighted to find him sleeping under the box-woods at the house. Eventually, my fears subsided because Chaucer's heart was home.

It was worth all the effort just to have my dogs sitting on my driveway, wagging their tails. It was not their work that I wanted; it was their devotion. Is their devotion helpful to me? No—it is a pain! They bark at the wrong people, and they don't bark when they need to be barking. I cannot keep Virginia from jumping all over guests. Both dogs fight over my attention and knock my hands with their heads to get me to pet them every day. Virginia and Chaucer even steal cat food from my cats, Dr. Pepper and Puss-n-Boots.

The fact is that they are trouble, but I love them and feel I would die if I lost their devotion. Has God made my cats to just sit around, priss around, and be pretty worthless? Well, maybe to someone who is not their master, but to their master whose windowsill they sit on, those prissy, sleepy cats are useless but *priceless!*

Now, if I have that much love for my dogs and cats and that much jealousy to have their devotion, think about how God feels toward us! Having an object that is devoted to you is priceless. God was so willing to gather a group of people together who are purely devoted just to Him, He sacrificed His only Son. This was worse than dying a thousand deaths, but our Father went through all of this pain to find those who are really devoted—the genuine articles. Have we embarrassed God in front of Satan, as Chaucer did me in front of the horse trainer? Can't God even get you to come home and leave the food behind for a few minutes? Who wants a dog that's devoted to the next-door neighbors and barks at you when you drive in your driveway? Could it be that we are devoted to the food and barking at God? I'm afraid a few of us are. Are we staying home long enough to let Him show us that He is the loving Master?

We should be devoted to God and barking at the food. We should be devoted to our spouses and barking at others who are trying to snare us. We should be devoted to our employers

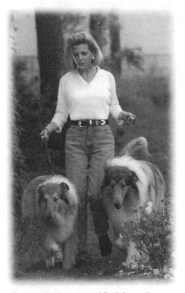

Gwen with her dogs, Virginia and Chaucer

and barking at some employee who is trying to get us off track with our devotion. We should be honoring the parents who brought us into the world and teachers who are trying to get us on the right path, and rejecting the peers who try to make us undevoted to those in authority.

COMING HOME FOR GOOD

How could Chaucer come home for good? Symbolically, how can you get to the point that you no longer desire more food, more money, sexual relations outside marriage, or any praise other than God's praise? Believe me, you can! There is a Promised Land! How do you know you will be set free from the desire to eat the second half of the hamburger if your body is not calling for it? Because once you love God, you cannot love another—so you cannot love food at the same time. Just as the barn no longer calls Chaucer, food will no longer call your name.

Actually, the horse trainer still calls to Chaucer, and the number three combo is still calling your name when you drive by. The world will always be out there. But since you hear only the voice of the One you love, you no longer hear the world's voice! If you do, your devotion is in the wrong place. If you are listening only to God when the pan of brownies calls your name from the pantry tonight, you won't hear that food. You'll be off sharing your day with God, listening to the voice of the One you really love. When the number three combo calls your name as you drive home, it will be like the wind blowing.

I am not a wonderful, competent, intelligent prize, but I am devoted, and I adore God, and that is the supreme good— the meaning and the purpose of setting our hearts into motion.

Instead, you'll find yourself listening to God singing a love song to you on the radio. You will hear the voice of the One you love. "My sheep listen to my voice," Jesus said (John 10:27a).

That's not to say that you will never be tempted by food again. I advise you to have a healthy fear of running back to the barn too many times. God hurts and eventually becomes angry, and He can allow you to die in the arms of Egypt if that's what you want. It is difficult to rebuild trust in a child who has continually slipped out the window at night to hang around with hoodlums. It's difficult to really depend upon a spouse who has broken your heart with an affair. It's awkward to rebuild faith in an employee who has a pattern of being more loyal to self or to another employee. But more important, you have to understand that it is difficult for God to trust us when we have had previous horizontal relationships or idols. So, I'm telling you: work out your own saving relationship with fear and trembling, as it says in Philippians 2:12. You need to sell everything, so to speak, to get this relationship back in good shape.

It scares me to think what would have happened to Chaucer had I not stepped in when I did. And I've got to admit, there was a point in the weeks of work with Chaucer that I wondered if I would ever see his heart home again. But I did. If Chaucer can do it, so can you!

If you are trying to build a relationship with God, then you must stay home. That is what God is trying to accomplish through the desert. He's bringing you to a point where you cannot avoid going to Him for what you need. You're leashed up, just as I had to leash Chaucer and Virginia. I made sure they had water and some dry dog food, but they were going to have to stay in their backyard. In most deserts, we can't go to the credit card because the credit card is full, and we can't get advice from anyone because God won't allow it to be any good. In my case, I couldn't go to excessive alcohol because I was already a thin eater and it made me sick, and I didn't even know what a drug dealer looked like. I had no one else to turn to but God. I was leashed up. That's how our coordinated God works. Every time I would go to His Word, He would show me that man does not live on bread alone, but on every word that comes from the mouth of the Lord. And He would speak to me first one way, then another.

LOVE IS THE ANSWER

The desert wanderings worked on me. I began to love His ideas more than my own ideas. And now, no matter who I am with, I am always talking with God. God is my very best friend, my comfort, my praise, my source of money, and my source of food. He is my heart's love. I am not a wonderful, competent, intelligent prize, but I am devoted, and I adore God, and that is the supreme good—the meaning and the purpose of setting our hearts into motion. Being devoted is not a work—it should be a natural characteristic of our personality. Being devoted to God is essential if we are expecting answered prayers, for-giveness, and salvation.

God coordinated and arranged everything to plant your heart that was created to love Him in His desert and to prepare for His kingdom. Just like a flower, once planted, your heart will grow and blossom.

But if it is uprooted, it will die. If your heart has wandered from your marriage, you need to stay home and focus on the spouse God has given you. If your heart has wandered as an employee, you need to stay home, so to speak, with your boss and focus on meeting his or her needs. If your heart has wandered from obeying and honoring your parents, you need to stay home and rebuild that relationship. Stay home, stay focused, stay in or under this authority, stay in the desert with God, and you will wake up in the Promised Land!

You may not feel very loving or feel loved. Let me tell you: you are loved. God's creation in general lets you know you are treasured. When my cat turns loving circles around me, it warms my heart to give him a bowl of milk. How much more does God adore you and want to shower you with what you want when you turn loving circles around Him? A lot more! As we learned from the plagues, He will fight for your love and devotion!

I think I have figured out one of the reasons that some people feel at arm's length and stay at arm's length from God. Take a moment and read Jesus' parable of the four soils in Matthew 13:3–8. Some seed fell on the rock, and then some seed fell on soil that was thin with rock underneath. The seed is God's love—His kingdom of love. The soil is a heart of man and the rock is a heart of hate, the antithesis of love. Love cannot root in hate. The second heart had some ability to respond to the love, but because hate, malice, jealousy, and anger were solidly fixed in the heart, love could not take root. The third soil was a heart of love—but it also loved the world—but it loved God—but it also loved the world. Where the heart is divided, the world will always win out.

FEAST ON JESUS CHRIST

You must believe in God. Repent from these behaviors that are the antithesis of belief in God, and then grow in love. Practically, how do you do that? You focus on God and on His teachings and on the love

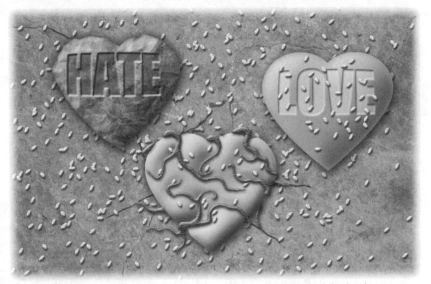

God's kingdom of love cannot take root in a heart of hate, and it cannot thrive in a heart choked by the love of this world.

of Jesus Christ. You immerse yourself in God's ways. You baptize yourself into the likeness of Jesus Christ.

Yes, the answer is to focus on Jesus, but I'm warning you very strongly to watch out for Satan's latest attack on God's church. Satan is resigned to the fact that the church is going to preach "focus on Jesus," so his method of attack is to make you focus on the externals of Jesus, not His pure-hearted, sacrificial, selfless, and undying passionate love for the Father. For example, Satan will work through false teachers who describe a Jesus who disciplined Himself for the Father and tell you that the application to your life should be that you get up early every morning to have a regimented quiet time with God. Remember that Satan will try to produce counterfeits. What better way to do it than by a false prophet who says, "Focus on Christ," but then comes out with a subtle picture of a military sergeant who is highly disciplined, constantly fasting, and always driven and serious-minded—a son of God who denies himself everything and endorses only rustic lifestyles, sandals, and beards? Jesus was described by the people as a glutton and a drunkard (Matt. 11:18–19). I'm sure He wasn't a glutton or a drunkard, but He obviously enjoyed God's bountiful creation. Many of God's sheep know that something is missing in their lives, so they grab onto the false prophets, who at least have a plan. On the other end of the spectrum of false teachers are those who emphasize a Jesus who says to the prostitute, "Neither do I condemn you," and they leave out the expected command, which appears in the same verse, "Go now and leave your life of sin" (John 8:11). The Jesus we must focus on is the One who expected repentance or we would perish (Luke 13:3).

If you follow the false teachers, in the beginning you will get psyched up, but then you will not be able to keep it up. The result is that you feel like a failure. It is the same cycle as man-made dieting.

Do not diet, but eat naturally. Do not regiment a relationship. Look at me: I eat naturally with hunger and fullness and what my body calls for. I have a natural, respectful relationship with God that comes easily. It should be no different from growing in a relationship with your spouse. You just get to know him. Does your spouse make you memorize verses about him or read rule books about what he likes? No! You spend time with him, and because your heart is into it, you learn easily and quickly what he likes and doesn't like. He knows when your heart is not into it—and so does God.

I let my Bible fall open, following my heart and God's leading. I look for God's handiwork and ideas everywhere. I pray on my knees when I'm moved to do so. I talk to Him all the time. I sing songs of appreciation constantly. I laugh with Him if I think He is joyful, and I cry with Him if I think He is hurting. I do this because I want to do this. I do this because I love Him. It's easy!

My heart is so full of love that love spills over to my husband, my children, and my employees, and I feel the capacity to love you. That's how I know that God has love to spare—overflowing, abundant rivers and seas of love! My relationship with God is natural because I haven't left Him standing outside my door. I've let Him in and allowed Him to sit on the throne of my heart, which is exactly where He belongs, and I have submitted my body (His temple) to His services. This is appropriate. First Corinthians 3:16 states, "Don't you know that you yourselves are God's temple and that God's Spirit lives in you?"

So when you focus on Jesus, focus on His natural love relationship with God. By imitating that, you will grow in love with God, and don't let any false teachers tell you any different. Jesus said, "If you loved me, you would be glad that I am going to the Father, for the Father is greater than I" (John 14:28b).

For you who are falling out of love with food and into love with God, out of love with the medicine cabinet, cigarettes, or alcohol and into love with God, for you who are now getting this loving feeling from God and are no longer running to sexual lusts or perverted sexual habits, let your heart be at peace. Do not let Satan ever rob you of your joy because nothing can come between you and this love for God when your heart cries, "Abba, Father." Now that you know that your heart cannot love two things, don't let Satan's false accusations burden you. And no longer live in fear that you are not good enough because perfect love of God casts out all fear. Just love—simply love—and you can feel it when you love God, and you can see it in your actions. The world and the things of the world do not matter to you anymore.

You Do Not Have to Be a Spiritual Superstar

Remember what it looks like to have a crush on someone. I have a crush on the Father, and this is what it looks like: I dress for Him and say, "God, do You like this outfit?" I get up in the night when I feel He is waking me, or early morning when He calls my name, because I hear the voice of the One I love, even if it is not physically audible. All other voices just fade away. I used to hide chocolate, but now I secure my *Bible* instead of my chocolate. I look forward to a rendezvous with God. I love reading about God and about Jesus Christ, who saved us and opened the door to heaven. I sing songs to Him all the time. No matter who I'm talking to, He is always on my mind. I can't take my eyes off Him now.

This isn't the behavior of a spiritual superstar. You have this same behavior right now, even though it may be directed toward something else. Perhaps you can identify with me. If you cannot, you can change right now. Jesus showed us the path, and it is easy to return to the path. Jesus told us this story about the father and the son who was not a spiritual superstar: "The son said to him, 'Father, I have sinned against heaven and against you. I am no longer worthy to be called your son.' But the father said to his servants, 'Quick! Bring the best robe and put it on him. Put a ring on his finger and sandals on his feet. Bring the fattened calf and kill it. Let's have a feast and celebrate. For this son of mine was dead and is alive again!'" (Luke 15:21–24a).

So God is saying to everyone now: "Quick!" And immediately, you will be celebrating. You could be celebrating with God right now. When you are throwing your heart toward the Father and adoring Jesus, you will grow in confidence of God's love for you. Never hesitate to ask for God's assurance. God's beloved David would get up in the mornings and look for God's unfailing love. As he said in Psalm 143:8a, "Let the morning bring me word of your unfailing love, for I have put my trust in you." Since my twenties, whenever I have needed God's reassurance, I have asked Him to send a sign. Answered prayers have built my faith so much. But when I'm feeling down and need to be reassured of God's love, I call out to Him in all sorts of ways. Here is one such story.

THE STORY OF THE SONG

One night my family went out to eat, and I remembered that I needed to pick up a gift certificate at a music store. The whole family went with me to the music store, and the kids said they wanted to get a CD, and then my husband, David, said that he might get a good CD, so I prayed to the Lord, "God, if there is something You want me to have in this huge, wide store, please guide me to it."

I'm not very good with names of musicians or groups or songs. We had only about three or four albums at my house when I was really young. I think one of them was *Color Me Barbra* by Barbra Streisand and one was Herb Alpert and the Tijuana Brass with *A Taste of Honey*. And another one was Gary Lewis and the Playboys. I haven't even seen these albums in almost twenty years.

While I was looking around the store, my eyes fell on the old Gary Lewis album, and I recognized one of the songs, "This Diamond Ring." So I bought the CD, and I was so proud of my little selection—until we got back into the car to compare our purchases. My family humiliated me so badly that I just left the CD in the sack on the floor of my car for several days. On the way home, we listened to David's purchase, Cat Stevens's *Teaser and the Firecat*.

As the week went by, God put me through several tests, and I felt that life was too hard. It seemed as if I had been abandoned, but I could feel my own devotion to God. Was He rejecting my devotion? Early one morning, I got down on my knees in front of my sunrise window and cried out to God to give me a clear, clear sign that He was with me. I asked God specifically: "Do You love me, or are You upset with me? Please show me that You are in love with me!" I told Him I didn't care what sign He sent. I just needed it to really hit my heart.

Well, nothing happened immediately, so I went about my regular routine. I got dressed, fed the dogs, and was running a little behind. When I got in the car, I felt compelled to do something unusual for me. Usually, I just get in the car, hardly putting on my seat belt, and take off. But that morning, I just had to put the Gary Lewis CD into the CD player. I was unfamiliar with CDs, so it was a real task to even get the seal wrap off. I was so driven to get into this CD case that I even broke a fingernail trying to open it.

I finally got it open and figured out how to load the CD into the player, and I was on my way out the driveway. I must have hit the third track accidentally because for the first time, God was singing back to me the love song I had been singing to Him for twenty years. I had forgotten this simple little song, "Save Your Heart for Me," was by Gary Lewis and the Playboys.

I cried the whole way to work, playing the song over and over. Not only had God answered my prayer while I was in the music store that day, but He had answered my prayer that morning in a powerful way.

He is singing a song for you, too. He does not reject anyone who wants this salvation of a devoted love. God's heart is here, hovering over the face of the people, waiting for you to direct your devotion toward the best-looking, most-coordinated, best-warrior and most-able-to-save-you God of the universe. He deserves your heart—give it to Him. Don't let the stars get in your eyes. Save your heart for Him.

What You Can Do Today

⧜ *Go where God is leading you in Scripture.*

⧜ *Think about the people in authority over you.* How can each relationship teach you something about your relationship with God and His authority?

⧜ *Recall a specific time when you felt the pain of rejection.* Now, with that perspective, think about God's pain when He—the Creator of the universe—gets rejected for a bowl of chips and dip! Commit yourself to loving God more than the food, and offer God your devotion instead of the sting of rejection.

⧜ *Turn your face toward the Creator.* Think about Chaucer and Virginia and their misplaced devotion. Are you barking at God when you should be barking at the extra food? When you feel tempted, bark at the worldly temptation that is trying to turn you away from God.

⧜ *Be willing to be used.* You've read about the four soils—the four types of hearts. Which soil are you? Make this story real for you, and make your heart the soft, nurturing soil that is willing to be moved in any way that the Master Planter desires.

_____

_____

_____

_____

_____

_____

_____

_____

_____

Take Me to the Movies

As soon as I get to the movie theater, I can smell the popcorn and the hot dogs. I like to make sure I am hungry when I arrive, so most of the time I won't eat supper before going to the movies. (If I've eaten supper, I skip the movie snacks.) If I'm good and hungry, my first stop is the concession stand. First, I rate the choices available to me. I scan the sweets, the salty snacks, the popcorn, and the drinks. Then I make my selection: usually some salty popcorn with extra butter and a diet drink—and lots of napkins. Sometimes I also pick up some peanut M&Ms. Once we all find what we like, we find a comfortable seat and start to enjoy our snacks. I find the best kernels of popcorn with just the right amount of butter and salt on them. I like to eat one kernel at a time so I can savor the combined flavors of the popcorn, salt, and butter. I also sip from my diet drink between bites. I alternate my sips and bites until I have had enough salt. Keep in mind that I still have my box of candy, so I do not want to fill up entirely on the popcorn. When I have finished with the popcorn, I take another sip from my diet drink before I begin my sweet snack. If the candy comes in a variety of colors or flavors, I will eat my favorite colors and flavors first. I take a bite, savor it, and take a sip from my diet drink. After the movie is over, I discard the rest of the popcorn because it is just no longer appealing. Since movie candy usually comes in a box, it is easy to close the lid and take the rest home to enjoy at another time. A night out at the movies makes for a wonderful evening—if the movie is any good, that is! Remember, God goes with you everywhere, even the movies!

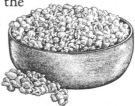

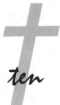

ten

CLOUD AND FIRE

We have read about the terrifying plagues that God brought upon Egypt. Through the wind, the rain, lightning, and hail—through a river of blood, a swarm of insects—through supernatural power and even death itself, Satan and all the world saw that God and God alone was the One to worship. God displayed superior power and superior intellect. He confirmed that He is the God of creation and the King of kings, and He demonstrated His rightful position as the one true God of the universe. God commanded that this story be told from generation to generation because the message is foundational. Our God is the God of theatrics and drama, of parables, mysteries, and wonders. He is the God who created and used the earth as a theater and a backdrop to explain His relationship with mankind. God is indeed alive and is indeed the very large force creating and controlling the elements of the earth. He shook the earth to release the hold that the world had on the heart of man. He showed all nations that He was more powerful than the earth and its hold. Mankind would never have to wonder again whether the world of food and other secret loves has more power than the God of the universe. God indeed has all the power!

MARRIAGE IN A DESOLATE AREA

The plagues, the Exodus, and the display of God's power sound like a good place to end this romantic, heroic rescue story. But it is not the end—it is the *beginning*. It is the beginning of a marriage between you and God in a desolate area. We have all traveled on a long spiritual journey, parallel to that of the Israelites, to get to the point where we are now. We have had a parallel exodus from our slavery and strongholds. By now we have tasted the heavy testing of the desert, and either we have understood it or we are stuck in some sand pit up to our necks. This desert is no ordinary testing. It is very heavy, and I know your pain. God gives us only what we can bear, and He knows your pain.

This familiar passage from Romans 8:38–39 states, "For I am convinced that neither death nor life, neither angels nor demons, neither the present nor the future, nor any powers, neither height nor depth, nor anything else in all creation, will be able to separate us from the love of God that is in Christ Jesus our Lord."

If God loves us this much, why in the world don't we recognize it? Well, the problem is that we have totally redefined *love* so that we can't even identify it. And we have a generation of parents and children coming up who don't even know what it looks like. In this chapter, we will reexamine the true definition of *love*.

The Bible helps us find the path that will lead us straight to the heart of the Father. It helps us to circumvent the mountains and valleys, and it provides street lamps for dark paths. It will help us avoid the dreadful parts of the desert that are thirsty and waterless, and it will help us avoid the scorpions, snakes, sand pits, and desert storms. If we do not honor His precepts and stay in His Word, shouting it from the street corners, writing it on the doorposts, and talking about it when we are going in and coming out—then my friends, we might retrace some of the wicked desert paths that the Israelites walked.

In 1 Corinthians, the Apostle Paul wrote warnings based upon Israel's walk in the desert and told the early Christians the following: "Nevertheless, God was not pleased with most of them; their bodies were scattered over the desert. Now these things occurred as examples to keep us from setting our hearts on evil things as they did. . . . These things happened to them as examples and were written down as warnings for us, on whom the fulfillment of the ages has come" (1 Cor. 10:5–6, 11). These words are as important today as they were when Paul first gave them to the early Christians.

THE HEART OF MAN MUST BE CONTINUALLY WARNED

Why do we have to be warned? Because we are weak. We were made weak so that our hearts would have the flexibility and sensitivity to respond. Our hearts were made with a tenderness so that the Spirit of God could penetrate and permeate them, but this weakness leaves the heart of man vulnerable to other spirits.

Even if you have lost all your excess weight and totally laid your stronghold down, your candle must remain burning. We are a light. The book of Luke says, "No one lights a lamp and puts it in a place where it will be hidden. . . . Instead he puts it on a stand. . . . See to it, then, that the light within you is not darkness" (11:33, 35). So we are to *see to it*, which is an active examining process for our ever-vulnerable and tender hearts. And that is why we have been warned.

BEYOND THE EXODUS

For those seeking true love, we must start with Israel's history—the history that lies beyond the mighty Exodus. The Bible tells us that after the plagues, "the Israelites set out from Rameses on the fifteenth day of the first month, the day after the Passover. They marched out boldly in full view of all the Egyptians, who were burying all their firstborn, whom the LORD had struck down" (Num. 33:3–4a). Once they were across the Red Sea, there was much singing and dancing. The celebration was great. Miriam, Moses' sister, led all the women in dance and song before the Lord (Ex. 15:20–21). Egypt—that is, the earth—was exposed for what it was: defenseless, worthless, and resourceless. Not one child of God wanted to stay in the man-made civilization of the mighty Egypt. No, they all chose to follow God, no matter where it led them . . . or at least that's what they thought.

The mighty plagues shook the earth more than three thousand years ago, and God is shaking the earth today to loosen the idols of our hearts. Now, the shaking of God we have endured. The Exodus we have endured. In fact, God says, "You yourselves have seen what I did to Egypt and how I carried you on eagles' wings and brought you to Myself." But are we enduring the fire of the desert? The early desert travelers did not.

I know this is the ultimate testing ground because of the weary and defeated desert travelers I have seen. I've seen plenty of hearts spring up and respond to the love of the Lord and grow in love toward the Father. But when God's hot sun comes out, they wither. When the heart is tested, only the root of *true* love will flourish.

The Israelites accepted the Exodus but despised the desert. The root of a plant is the tap line to the deep water and nourishment of life. Without a root we have no water. The hot sun of the desert is the most intense part of our journey with the Father. Heat is the only test for true love and rebellion. How much heat was God applying to the Israelites in this desert that a whole generation of people would not be rooted deeply enough to endure the trials? What kind of test is God putting us through today that the writer of Hebrews would express so graphically God's warnings?

> *Today, if you hear his voice,*
> *do not harden your hearts*
> *as you did in the rebellion,*
> *during the time of testing in the desert,*
> *where your fathers tested and tried me*
> *and for forty years saw what I did.*

That is why I was angry with that generation,
      and I said, "Their hearts are always going astray,
      and they have not known my ways."
So I declared on oath in my anger,
      "They shall never enter my rest." (Heb. 3:7b–11)

The writer went on to warn them:

See to it, *brothers, that none of you has a sinful, unbelieving heart that*
turns away from the living God. But encourage one another daily,
as long as it is called Today, so that none of you may be hardened by
sin's deceitfulness. We have come to share in Christ if we hold firmly
till the end *the confidence we had at first. As has just been said:*

      "Today, if you hear his voice,
            do not harden your hearts
      as you did in the rebellion."

Who were they who heard and rebelled? Were they not all those Moses
led out of Egypt? And with whom was he angry for forty years? Was
it not with those who sinned, whose bodies fell in the desert? And to
whom did God swear that they would never enter his rest if not to
those who disobeyed? So we see that they were not able to enter,
because of their unbelief. Therefore, since the promise of entering his
rest still stands, let us be careful that none of you be found to
have fallen short of it. (Heb. 3:12–4:1, emphasis added)

Can we still today make the same mistakes that the Israelites
did? What went wrong after the Exodus? What emotions did these
rescued followers feel to be so rebellious? Did they feel abandoned?
Did they feel unloved? Did they have no fear of God? Was there an
absence of true love in their hearts? Well, we must follow the
ancients into the desert to find out this mystery.

DESERT RESPONSE JOURNEY

After the Exodus, the delivered Israelites were on the edge of the desert, climbing down off the mighty Eagle's wings (Ex. 19:4) and waiting to start their "Desert Response Journey." After the rescue, this mighty Warrior decided to present Himself in the form of a protective, caring cloud. It was a cloud to guide them by day, and the cloud never left its place over the people (Ex. 13:21–22). The Bible tells us that the Lord looked down from the pillar of cloud and the glory of the Lord appeared in the cloud, which showed the continual care and good pleasure of the Lord. Scripture tells us that God would peek over the side of this heavenly mist and look at His people. Sometimes, the cloud would lower, so that He could hear what His precious lambs were saying. The cloud also provided a "shelter and shade from the heat of the day, and a refuge and hiding place from the storm and rain" (Isa. 4:6).

The care did not end at sunset. At dusk, God turned the cloud into a pillar of fire so that it could be seen against the backdrop of the navy blue night.

The care did not end at sunset. At dusk, God turned the cloud into a pillar of fire so that it could be seen against the backdrop of the navy blue night. As a night-light is to a frightened child, God ensured the most loving care by supplying this glorious pillar of fire at night so that He could guide them and protect them in the darkness. No worries for the children of God. Whenever the cloud and the fire lifted from above the tent, the Israelites set out; whenever the cloud settled, the Israelites encamped. The cloud and fire remained over the tabernacle day and night, always within sight of all the house of Israel during their travels (Num. 9:17–23). Along with the cloud by day and the fire by night, God sent an angel to travel in front of Israel's army (Ex. 14:19).

As you can see, the children of God were guided completely. Since the cloud hovered over them with protection and concern, and sheltered them from the storm and rain, how could anyone's heart rebel with this backdrop of care from the Father? And as you might have guessed, nothing went wrong for two straight days! But by day three, things were not okay.

Desert Test Number 1

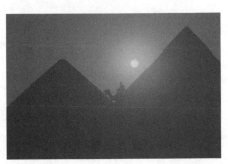

"Moses led Israel from the Red Sea and they went into the Desert of Shur. For three days they traveled in the desert without finding water. When they came to Marah, they could not drink its water because it was bitter. . . . So the people grumbled against Moses, saying, 'What are we to drink?'" (Ex. 15:22–24). Then Moses cried out to the Lord for help! Does it seem to be a fair and innocent question to you? "What are we to drink?" Remember, they are only three days past the theatrical, supernatural Exodus and only three days into the testing, and they are already criticizing, faultfinding, nagging, and muttering— basically, questioning the ability and leadership of the great CEO of the universe. Just three days without knowing how God was going to supply them with water. Three days of having to use faith. Three days past the Exodus, and the heart of man was mad at God. I am sure that they had a supply of liquids in their water bags. They just had nothing concrete in front of them at that moment to assure them of the water for tomorrow. Their discomfort, at that moment, was just in their minds.

This group of people had no idea that this romantic Savior would purposely, knowingly lead them into suffering, pain, and hardship, especially within seventy-two hours of leaving Egypt. Why would a God want you for His own and then take you to a graveyard? The problem of this generation is the same problem that we have today. We have redefined *love* to the point that we don't even recognize it when it slaps us in the face. The Israelites knew little about love, so little that they didn't expect that God would intentionally take them to the verge of death again and again to help them build trust in Him and faith in His ability—in other words, to learn love. That *is* love, whether you recognize it or not. And they didn't recognize it, so they kept screaming to Moses, "Why did you take us out of Egypt and into the desert to die?"

Their failure to recognize love wasn't going to stop God from exercising its true definition. The Lord took them to the brink of death and then delivered them. God showed Moses a piece of wood to throw into the water to make the water become sweet. Then God led them to Elim, where there were twelve springs of water—not just one, but twelve—and seventy palm trees (Ex. 15:25a, 27).

God's heart seemed to cry out, "Now trust Me! Remember the plagues. Recall the parting water. Drink of the twelve springs of water. And learn to love and trust Me!"

The Lord calmly handled these first signs of ignorance from His children. He wanted them to know what His purpose for them was and how much He loved them. He wanted them to understand that the desert-then-oasis combination was a series of testing-then-reward that He was going to put them through. He would lead them to the edge of death in the desert and then immediately to deliverance, or a symbolic oasis. This desert-oasis combination would happen again and again so that the children of God would have no fear of physical death, have great faith in God, and again build a love relationship with this mighty Lover, Warrior, Defender, and Supplier.

God had seen with a broken heart that the powerful display of the plagues had not even dented the heart of man, and that the parting of the Red Sea had not even penetrated the belief of man. But perhaps the twelve springs of water and the seventy palm trees would be the final education the people would need to understand that life and love come from death to their wills and trust in God's suffering. Let's continue deeper into the barren desert to see if that was so.

Desert Test Number 2

After they camped at the massive oasis, "the whole Israelite community set out from Elim and came to the Desert of Sin, which is between Elim and Sinai, on the fifteenth day of the second month after they had come out of Egypt" (Ex. 16:1).

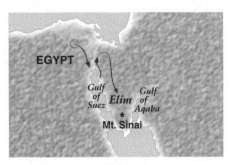

In this desert test, they weren't thirsty; they were hungry: "In the desert the whole community grumbled against Moses and Aaron. The Israelites said to them, 'If only we had died by the LORD's hand in Egypt! There we sat around pots of meat and ate all the food we wanted, but you have brought us out into this desert to starve this entire assembly to death!'" (Ex. 16:2–3).

They had just had the thirst deprivation test followed by twelve springs of water in the middle of the desert. It was no ordinary oasis. God supplied big time. But just a few days later, God tried the food deprivation test, and the children of God, with no trust, no patience, and in a spoiled way, griped back to Moses and the Lord. Once again, like the mother with a crying baby, the Lord jumped to please the spoiled Israelites and said to Moses, "I will rain down bread from heaven for you. The people are to go out each day and gather enough for that day" (Ex. 16:4a).

The bread that the Israelites called manna was abundant. It appeared out of nowhere, like the dew on the morning grass, miraculous and prolific. They did not have to work for it, and they were not to gather more than they needed for the day. God was trying hard to teach them to trust in His ability to supply. So again: thirst, and then water provided in a excellent way. Hunger, and then food provided in a heavenly way.

Now perhaps they understood the definition of *love*. Perhaps now they were ready to trust and enjoy this stirring relationship—

a relationship of giving and guidance and of precious protection from the Father. A relationship out away from the slavery of earth and the hubbub of the world! A place where the root of love can grow deep and desert flowers can start to bloom. The basis for this love would have to be trust, so God's heart cried out again, "Please trust Me! I am a good God! I know what I'm doing with your heart! My healing is miraculous, and My salvation is sure. And there is nothing I wouldn't do to make you feel My love."

Desert Test Number 3

But not long after this event, the Israelites began Desert Test Number 3. The Bible states,

> The rabble with them began to crave other food, and again the Israelites started wailing and said, "If only we had meat to eat! We remember the fish we ate in Egypt at no cost—also the cucumbers, melons, leeks, onions and garlic. But now we have lost our appetite; we never see anything but this manna!" . . . Moses heard the people of every family wailing, each at the entrance to his tent. (Num. 11:4–6, 10)

The Israelites had forgotten that this meat had come at great cost! In fact, it cost them their freedom, and they were enslaved to what looked like free food, but they had forgotten that it was small pittance for the subjugation of their lives. And we will look back on our years of dieting and remember the "free" foods and the optional calories, and not remember the entire enslavement we had to fat grams and exercise programs.

When mankind doesn't know the definition of *love* and is feeding off physical food rather than spiritual food, the appetite is never satisfied. Numbers 11:10b tells us that God became *exceedingly angry*. The beloved children of God—the rescued, the well-watered, the well-fed—were now craving other food, more than they needed. It wasn't a simple request. It was a demand, coming once again from a generation who had no concept of what they had and a generation who couldn't recognize eternal love.

This problem just emphasizes the fact that we have redefined *love* and we have decided for God what love should look like. Anger and love run side by side. If God did not love and care deeply, then there would just be apathy. When you hear or read the words "God was angry" in the Bible, you should think of a dangerous jealousy—a passionate Lover who is ready to fight for the attention of His precious bride. Again, anger has been totally misinterpreted, and we ignore the "anger" passages in the Bible, thinking that that's the God of the Old Testament. How wrong! References to anger, judgment, and final warning are all over the New Testament because God still loves us as much as He did in the Old—it's simply a part of love. God's love for us has led to His jealousy, His anger, and His pain.

> *When mankind doesn't know the definition of love and is feeding off physical food rather than spiritual food, the appetite is never satisfied.*

> *If we deliberately keep on sinning after we have received the knowledge of the truth, no sacrifice for sins is left, but only a fearful expectation of judgment and of raging fire that will consume the enemies of God. Anyone who rejected the law of Moses died without mercy on the testimony of two or three witnesses. How much more severely do you think a man deserves to be punished who has trampled the Son of God under foot, who has treated as an unholy thing the blood of the covenant that sanctified him, and who has insulted the Spirit of grace? For we know him who said, "It is mine to avenge; I will repay," and again, "The Lord will judge his people." It is a dreadful thing to fall into the hands of the living God. (Heb. 10:26–31)*

There is a verse I came across in the book of Genesis when I was writing this chapter, and it said, "The LORD was grieved that he had made man on the earth, and his heart was filled with pain" (Gen. 6:6). His heart was *filled* with pain. And when a heart as big as God's is filled with pain, it's a *lot* of pain. In fact, this is no ordinary sensation that can be dismissed with aspirin or painkillers. And who is there to dry the tears of our heavenly Father?

When God heard the cries of these unpolished objects of His affection, He responded to them just as we do to our spoiled children. We do the knee-jerk response. We give the children anything that they want to stop the whining!

God told Moses to tell the people to get ready because He was going to provide meat for everyone the next day. Well, even Moses was shortsighted and said to the Lord: "Here I am among six hundred thousand men on foot, and you say, 'I will give them meat to eat for a whole month!' Would they have enough if flocks and herds were slaughtered for them? Would they have enough if all the fish in the sea were caught for them?" (Num. 11:21–22).

We rarely give God the credit He deserves. Very few people see all of His resources, His power, His coordination, and His genius. God was begging, "Why don't you just trust in Me?" Without this trust, we can never build the love.

"The LORD answered Moses, 'Is the LORD's arm too short? You will now see whether or not what I say will come true for you.' . . . Now a wind went out from the LORD and drove quail in from the sea. It brought them down all around the camp to about three feet above the ground, as far as a day's walk in any direction" (Num. 11:23, 31). And the quail kept coming and coming for hours on end: "All that day and night and all the next day the people went out and gathered quail. No one gathered less than ten homers [sixty bushels]. . . . But while the meat was still between their teeth and before it could be consumed, the anger of the LORD burned against the people, and he struck them with a severe plague" (Num. 11:32a, 33).

The pattern has been drought and then twelve springs of water—and no punishment. Hunger and then manna—more than could be consumed in great amounts daily—and no punishment. Finally, cravings above and beyond the need of man, resulting in meat up to their waists—but, this time, *with* punishment. It has moved from a desert-and-oasis combination of testing to a desert-and-oasis-*and-punishment* combination because mankind could not see or comprehend the love of God. And since God is love, He houses the definition of *love.* But man's prideful heart believed that it had a better definition of love than the Almighty God of the universe, and it just could not get God to repent.

Desert Test Number 4

The cloud of God remained over the tent. So God did not give up on the experiment on the heart of man to see if man would ever accept His definition of *love.* The next desert exam of God through Moses came from the Desert of Sin. At that location, there was no water for the people to drink. Does this test sound familiar? Not to the children of God. They see no correlation to the last "no-water-to-drink" test. They do not seem to remember anything. Just like the Israelites, we can be slow and very stubborn.

> *It has moved from a desert-and-oasis combination of testing to a desert-and-oasis-and-punishment combination because mankind could not see or comprehend the love of God.*

The forgetful, untrainable Israelites again quarreled with Moses, and this is what they said,

> "Give us water to drink!" Moses replied, "Why do you quarrel with me? Why do you put the LORD to the test?" But the people were thirsty for water there, and they grumbled against Moses. They said, "Why did you bring us up out of Egypt to make us and our children and livestock die of thirst?" Then Moses cried out to the LORD, "What am I to do with these people? They are almost ready to stone me!" The LORD

answered Moses, "Walk on ahead of the people. Take with you some
of the elders of Israel and take in your hand the staff with which you
struck the Nile, and go. I will stand there before you by the rock at
Horeb. Strike the rock, and water will come out of it for the people to
drink." So Moses did this in the sight of the elders of Israel. And he
called the place Massah and Meribah because the Israelites quar-
reled and because they tested the LORD saying, "Is the LORD among
us or not?" (Ex. 17:2b–8)

Let's dissect this question: "Is the LORD among us or not?" Now, I
don't think for one minute that the children of God failed to believe
that God existed—that was not the problem. Look at the Israelites'
question again: "Is God among us or not?" What could they possibly
be talking about? I believe that what the arrogant children of God
were saying was, "Is God with us or not?"—or better yet—"Is He
going to get with the program or not? He is either with us or against
us. Is God going to submit to our kingdom or not?" They had no use
for a God who was not going to serve their agenda. They were not
so sure that Jehovah was working out!

By the fourth test, the heat revealed that the state of the heart of
man was more unmanageable and unruly than first thought. These
were hearts that wanted God to repent if He was going to hang
around. The spoiled children always had a backup plan called
"Egypt" to run to if God didn't give them what they wanted! The
way they saw it, God would choose to let them rule, or they would
choose to return to Egyptian rule. People think so poorly of that horrible Satan who got kicked out of heaven because he wanted to rule
over God. Do we think we are any different? People who have not
yet submitted to God's leadership with food or other strongholds are
saying this very thing! It is still a struggle for power.

This problem is not new. Right now you may have a life that is
turned completely upside down, a home where the children rule the
parents. The parents are invited by the children to get with the pro-

gram or get out of their way. They completely manipulate the parents and use the parents. How does even a one-year-old know he can do this? Because the child can sense that the parent wants fellowship at almost any cost. The parent adores the child and the child adores himself—a nice combination for getting what you want. The parent jumps at the child's yelling or pouting. How difficult it is to discipline an object that you adore—and that has been God's dilemma all along!

We have all been around a spoiled child. If he would only submit, there would be peace and blessings on that child. Oh, but no. Temper tantrums, sarcasm, manipulation, anger, demands, and a tossing of the head are all you receive from the spoiled child. Could this be symbolic of how you treat God Almighty? It is extremely inappropriate to have the father or the mother bowing down to the child. If it were not for the parent, there would be no offspring. Yet the parent serves not only the needs, but also the whims of the *The spoiled children always had a backup plan called "Egypt" to run to if God didn't give them what they wanted!* spoiled child. How awkward to see the parent jumping for the son or daughter, or the owner of the business bowing down to the employees, or the husband bowing down to the wife, or the king serving the servants as they sit on the throne and demand more from the king. All of those pictures make me want to shout out: Improper! Immoral! Inappropriate! Unseemly! Proverbs 19:10 says, "It is not fitting for a fool to live in luxury—how much worse for a slave to rule over princes!"

The difference between the analogy of the parent-and-child relationship and the God-and-you relationship is that God would go to the ends of the earth for you. There is nothing that He wouldn't sacrifice and no amount of time that He wouldn't spend to win your embrace. There is nothing that He wouldn't do or hasn't done to make you experience His love. God had rescued His loved ones from His competitor. Man's tendency was to love the earth more than

God, so God beat up His competition and lured His beloved into the desert. However, He found that the desert brought forth another opponent: the god of self.

Is there anything in heaven above or on earth that would entice you to put yourself second? Have you tried to lose weight for your spouse, but you couldn't? You loved yourself more. Have you tried to lose weight for the sake of your children, so that they could see you live longer, but you saw that you loved yourself even more than your children? Well, could you do it for your parents? What about for God? Is there *anything* that could get you to put yourself second? I'm afraid the god of self reigns in many hearts.

The Israelites kept crying out, "Why have you brought us out of Egypt to die in the desert?" That's the point exactly: God brought them out to die—to die to their wills. But the desert only seemed to revive the will of man and make it stronger than it was while under the burden of slavery to the earth! The will of man was thriving, not dying as planned. Suffering in the desert was not killing the desire to rule. They still did not get that God is *God*.

But again, the cloud of God stayed over those rebellious hearts, patiently looking to see if anyone would consider joining His kingdom where He is the boss. What was the Father going to have to do? Throughout history, the heart of man has continued to have the same flaw. We welcome God when He does what we want, but we do not have any use for God if He goes against our wishes.

What was God going to do with His children to resolve this dilemma? How could He make it clear that He opposed their pride and their spoiled nature? No one is attracted to prideful people because they are so incredibly ignorant. It would not be honest of me to leave out the fact that God considered annihilation several times since none of His miraculous works seemed to penetrate the pride of man. Since He loved them too much and the pain was so great, He considered wiping them off the face of the earth. We have all seen desperate lovers.

How stupid that prideful people do not credit God for every move they make: their ability to walk, their ability to think, the beating of their hearts! God hates the ignorance of pride for good reason. No one is attracted to a spoiled child because that nature is repulsive. What was the Father to do?

Well, up to this point, nothing really drastic had happened to the children of God. There had been no major disciplining. It was almost as if God wanted to make completely sure that the line had been drawn in the sand. Surely, the grumbling and complaining were out of sheer ignorance of His love, for they had seen His force and could not deny that He was all-powerful; His commanding

The will of man was thriving, not dying as planned. Suffering in the desert was not killing the desire to rule. They still did not get that God is God.

performance of the plagues was not yet three months out of the picture. They saw the death angel cover the camp and the waters jump at His command. Just in case His power and His intentions were not understood, God gave them one more supernatural theatrical demonstration: Mount Sinai.

THE STORY OF MOUNT SINAI

God was hoping this would be the last display of power in an awesome manner and that it would solve the dilemma of ignorance and unrequited love in mankind. History, as recorded in Exodus, says,

> In the third month after the Israelites left Egypt—on the very day—
> they came to the Desert of Sinai. After they set out from Rephidim, they
> entered the Desert of Sinai, and Israel camped there in the desert in
> front of the mountain. . . . The LORD said to Moses, "I am going to come
> to you in a dense cloud, so that the people will hear me speaking with
> you and will always put their trust in you. . . . Go to the people and

*consecrate them today and tomorrow. Have them wash their clothes
and be ready by the third day, because on that day the LORD will come
down on Mount Sinai in the sight of all the people. Put limits for the
people around the mountain and tell them, 'Be careful that you do not
go up the mountain or touch the foot of it. Whoever touches the mountain shall surely be put to death.'"* (Ex. 19:1–2, 9–12)

The thought of meeting the Lord must have been ominous.
Finally, the time arrived. On the morning of the third day, it all
started. The sun was not shining as you might have imagined; the
birds were not singing. No, it was dark. Early in the morning, there
was a thick cloud over the mountain and great thunder and lightning, and a very loud trumpet blast. Everyone in the camp trembled.
Then Moses led the people out of the camp to meet with God, and
they stood at the foot of the mountain, and they knew to keep their
distance. Mount Sinai was covered with smoke because the Lord
descended on it in fire. The smoke billowed up from it like smoke
from a furnace, the whole mountain trembled violently, and the
sound of the trumpet grew louder and louder.

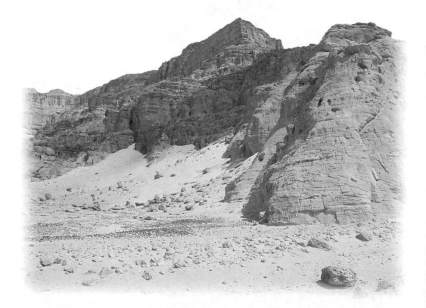

The Bible says,

> *When the people saw the thunder and lightning and heard the trumpet and saw the mountain in smoke, they trembled with fear. They stayed at a distance and said to Moses, "Speak to us yourself and we will listen. But do not have God speak to us or we will die." Moses said to the people, "Do not be afraid. God has come to test you, so that the fear of God will be with you to keep you from sinning."* (Ex. 20:18–20)

Even though that sounds like a strange statement—"don't be afraid"—it was God trying once more to wake up the inside force in the heart of man. However, He didn't want an outside force of fear to cause terror. That kind of fear doesn't invoke love. "Then the LORD said to Moses, 'Tell the Israelites this: "You have seen for yourselves that I have spoken to you from heaven: Do not make any gods to be alongside me; do not make for yourselves gods of silver or gods of gold"'" (Ex. 20:22–23).

Moses was on the mountain with God a long time, and when the people saw that Moses was so long in coming down from the mountain, they gathered around Aaron for a chance to take over, and they said, "Come, make us gods who will go before us. As for this fellow Moses who brought us up out of Egypt, we don't know what has happened to him" (Ex. 32:1b).

The thunder and the lightning and the supernatural trumpet sound and even the mountain moving by the voice of God did not deter the pride of man. They were ready to organize a coup to put man back in control.

Unfortunately, the right kind of fear that demands love, respect, and worship had not penetrated the heart of man at Mount Sinai. The thunder and the lightning and the supernatural trumpet sound and even the mountain moving by the voice of God did not deter the

pride of man. They were ready to organize a coup to put man back
in control.

They wanted a divine cloud that moved when they wanted to
move. So they built a golden calf from their gold earrings. And the
people bowed down to the idol and made sacrifices to it and said,
"These are your gods, O Israel, who brought you up out of Egypt"
(Ex. 32:8b).

Amazing! They were so arrogant that they thought that they
could create a god! The Israelites wanted to worship a robotic god,
not a real god. Likewise, anyone holding on to his idols or anyone
holding on to his food is waiting to worship a golden calf—a god that
will do his bidding.

While Moses was on the mountain, God looked down and saw
this awful behavior and told Moses to go away so that He could
just destroy the stiff-necked people (Ex.
32:9–10). God's heart was broken. But
Moses begged Him to rethink the situation for the sake of His own glory.

God knew that it was no more Mr. Nice Guy from that point on. He was finished with the little mountain chats. . . . This powder puff of a cloud would become a raging fire.

God knew clearly what He was up
against. Would He want to continue? Was
there hope for the soul of man? It was one
thing to expose Egypt for what it was—
worthless—but how would God convince
His people that He is more important than
the objects of His concern and affection?
How was He going to reverse the attitude
of the conniving child who knows how concerned God is and is taking advantage of it? How was He to convert the spoiled child?

God knew that it was no more Mr. Nice Guy from that point on.
He was finished with the little mountain chats. He was finished
with making sure that the rules were clear. This powder puff of a
cloud would become a raging fire. God had lost hope in His children.
He was ready to wipe them off the face of the earth. The price seemed

God led me to Weigh Down† to teach me that true joy and contentment lie in full surrender to Him. Learning to eat only when I was hungry and stopping when I was satisfied gave me an incredible sense of freedom. I noticed that the weight loss just happened as long as I was obedient, and the time with God was what I truly cherished.

Mike Sabourin—Northbridge, MA
Lost 100 lbs.
Has kept it off 3 years

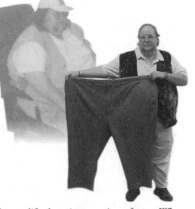

When my weight reached 500 pounds, I asked God to take my life or give me a new one. The next day God sent a friend who introduced me to Weigh Down†, and that was the beginning of my new life. Now, I've been off insulin for a year and a half and I'm continuing to lose weight. God is giving me many opportunities to share with others that He can also change their hearts and take them out of Egypt.

Randy Barker—Vallejo, CA
Lost 150 lbs.
. . . and losing!

Weigh Down† has been a life-changing experience for me. When I came to the program, I was miserable physically and struggling spiritually, with my weight at over 350 pounds. I soon learned how to replace food and the desire for food with the true and living God. I have now found freedom in ceasing my worship of food and building my relationship with the Lord.

Damon Cathey
Franklin, TN
Lost 95 lbs.
Has kept it off 2 years

At the age of 16, I found myself weighing 252 pounds, and I was told by my doctor that I would probably never weigh under 200 pounds. Well, here I am 90 pounds lighter, praise God! But the best thing that has happened is my renewed relationship with the Father.

Michael Sawvel—Wauseon, OH
Lost 90 lbs.

too high for true love, and nothing seemed to get through the heart of this adorable but maddening creature called man.

But Moses sought the favor of the Lord and tried to reason with God:

> *Why should your anger burn against your people, whom you brought out of Egypt with great power and a mighty hand? Why should the Egyptians say, "It was with evil intent that he brought them out, to kill them in the mountains and to wipe them off the face of the earth"? Turn from your fierce anger; relent and do not bring disaster on your people. Remember your servants Abraham, Isaac and Israel. (Ex. 32:11b–13a)*

God listened to Moses and did not completely annihilate His children.

All along, throughout the desert tests and pride-breaking events, the cloud remained above the camp. Mount Sinai was not the last place that God got angry on this desert journey.

One time the cloud came down, and God's heart got very close to the people. The Scripture says, "Now the people complained about their hardships in the hearing of the LORD, and when he heard them his anger was aroused" (Num. 11:1). He saw that they didn't like Him! "Then fire from the LORD burned among them and consumed some of the outskirts of the camp. When the people cried out to Moses, he prayed to the LORD and the fire died down. So that place was called Taberah, because fire from the LORD had burned among them" (Num. 11:1b–3).

The earth shook at the Exodus, and the earth shook at Mount Sinai. The cloud brought the people out of Egypt, and it never left them. Did the cloud and the fire and events of Mount Sinai penetrate the soul of man? I am afraid not. Most people died before they repented, and it was their children who entered the Promised Land. I hope this is not prophetic for this generation. God saw that His precious guidance from the cloud and fire was not enough light or love for mankind to be drawn to Him. Therefore, He was going to have to try one more time to get through the prideful shell and into the passionate love of the heart of man.

FROM CLOUD TO SPIRIT

When you look back on history, you would think that a low, hovering cloud would be near enough for the God of the universe to get through to the heart of man. But it was not. So one day, centuries after Mount Sinai, God decided to come closer to us than even a cloud. His word and His heart became flesh, and His own offspring came to earth and made His dwelling among us. Jesus Christ was full of grace and truth. He was closer than the pillar of fire and offered more than the shadow of the cloud. There was thunder in His footsteps, and there was lightning guidance in His words. And there was a fire of love for the Father, which was the light of all mankind: "Through him all things were made. . . . In him was life, and that life was the light of men. The light shines in the darkness, but the darkness has not understood it" (John 1:3–5).

The cloud of God was with His Son, and He gave great protection to Jesus' words so that the sheep of God would finally see His love, something that the Pharisees, the religious leaders in Jesus' day, had always distorted. As Jesus explained the message of dying to one's will through His baptism, the cloud of God opened and the Spirit of God descended on His Son as a dove (Matt. 3:16). That day, Jesus drove home a message of life-from-death that was better than the desert tests were ever able to do! And God was hopeful and said, "This is my Son, whom I love; with him I am well pleased" (Matt. 3:17).

As God looked down from the cloud, He saw His Son walk among men—He heard everything they said and saw their hearts. At the end of thirty-three years, the cloud grew very dark, darker than it had ever grown. The Bible tells us: "At the sixth hour darkness came over the whole land until the ninth hour" (Mark 15:33).

Remember, back in the desert with the Israelites, God had come close to the people and heard the real way they felt about Him. He heard. He got it. He got that the people really did not like Him or His ideas or His decisions. They had no trust in Him. They had no need for Him.

Centuries later, when He came even closer to man and walked with man for thirty-three years, He recognized the real truth about how man feels about Him. He acknowledged it. He accepted it—that we really hate Him and want Him to go away. The day God left His Son vulnerable to the heart of mankind, we murdered Him. We murdered Him, buried Him in the tomb, rolled a stone over it, and sealed His body inside. We tossed our heads in the desert and murdered His Son, who was the likeness of Himself. We killed God.

He is close to each of us now, and He sees how we're living. He has figured out whether we want Him around. We are not worthy of the hovering cloud of love and guidance that we have been given throughout the centuries. But God went one step farther. After the death of Christ, the cloud got even closer. Though we pushed Him away and murdered His Son, He turned His pure and shining face back toward us and embraced us by sending His Holy Spirit to the hearts that would repent and be baptized into His will.

Moreover, as the years have passed, God has left us a heavenly cloud of witnesses that are watching us daily to spur us on—Abel, Enoch, Noah, Abraham, Sarah, Isaac, Jacob, Joseph, Moses, David, and the prophets. Hebrews 12:1 says, "Therefore, since we are surrounded by such a great cloud of witnesses, let us throw off everything that hinders and the sin that so easily entangles, and let us run with perseverance the race marked out for us."

God has provided every opportunity for you to leave your pride, your self-love, your idols, and your strongholds behind. Come to this new covenant of love that is written in your heart. God is the One who deserves to warehouse all pride, yet He lowered Himself below you and me into death. He allowed Himself to be sealed in a tomb for our love.

Read this amazing reference to Mount Sinai in Hebrews 12:

You have not come to a mountain that can be touched and that is
burning with fire . . . to a trumpet blast or to such a voice speaking
words that those who heard it begged that no further word be spoken
to them, because they could not bear what was commanded: "If even
an animal touches the mountain, it must be stoned." The sight was so
terrifying that Moses said, "I am trembling with fear." But you have
come to Mount Zion, to the heavenly Jerusalem, the city of the living
God. You have come to thousands upon thousands of angels in joyful
assembly, to the church of the firstborn, whose names are written in
heaven. You have come to God, the judge of all men, to the spirits of
righteous men made perfect, to Jesus the mediator of a new covenant.
(vv. 18–24a)

Hebrews describes this new covenant as a mountain of hope, an
approachable mountain with thousands upon thousands of angels
surrounding it. It is a long way from
Mount Sinai. It is Mount Zion—the city of
the righteous—the city of the living God.
Instead of smoke and fire, it is a cloud of
love. Instead of death, it is life. Instead of a
trumpet blast, it is whispers of the righteous men made wholehearted in love with

> *Open your eyes and*
> *see God's angels*
> *surrounding you.*
> *God is crying out*
> *one more time.*

God. Instead of an untouchable mountain, it is an embracing Holy
Spirit. Instead of Moses and the tablets, it is Jesus Christ, the
Mediator of this loving covenant.

So what is true love? God's love from the Old Testament to the
New Testament has not changed. He has always had the firm, true
love that expects wholehearted devotion. When He brought His love
to earth in the flesh—through Jesus Christ—with a forgiveness system in which He took all the grief and did all the giving in, He
expected a response. So the prophetic voice of the book of Hebrews

warns us, "Today, if you hear his voice, do not harden your hearts as you did in the rebellion" (Heb. 3:7–8).

Please obey God, and when it seems difficult to wait for hunger, and if dying to your will seems too hard, cry out to God and wait for Him; and He will lift you up and reward you. Open your eyes and see God's angels surrounding you. God is crying out one more time, "Just trust Me to feed you. Let go of control."

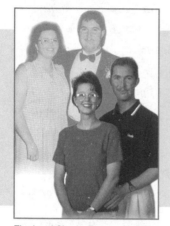

I have dieted off and on throughout my life with fat grams, calories, videos, etc., with short-term results. But the weight never stayed off. Then I heard of Weigh Down†. At first, there was only some weight loss because I didn't take it to the spiritual level. Then I went to a Weigh Down† class with my husband. I have lost 58 pounds so far, and Thad has dropped 45. We both feel so much better and constantly comment on how much more rewarding our lives are since we stopped worshiping food. When people ask how we've lost weight, I always tell them about Weigh Down† and about how wonderful our God is!
Thad & Shawn Duncan—Clayton, NC

Thad and Shawn Duncan find life much more rewarding since they've changed their focus from food to God.

What You Can Do Today

▰▰▰ *Go where God is leading you in Scripture.*

▰▰▰ *Trust in God.* In spite of all the things that He has already done for you, are there still times that you question His timetable or doubt His capability to provide for you? If so, commit yourself right now to stop demanding from God and questioning His abilities.

▰▰▰ *Demonstrate your trust in God.* Wait for hunger, and eat only when your God-given hunger mechanism cues you. Do not grab for *anything* that God has not provided for you.

▰▰▰ *Notice the warnings that God and Jesus give.* Because of His love for us, God offers many warnings in His Word and often gives us chance after chance to obey. Stop and ask yourself: What is God warning me about? How can I take heed and obey God's desire for me? And then thank the heavenly Father for His love and His concern for you.

▰▰▰ *Respectfully obey God's commands.* The Israelites were fearful at Mount Sinai. What kind of fear do you have of God? Are you afraid because you know you have been disobedient, or do you have the fear of God that will *keep* you from sinning? Our God is very powerful. Commit yourself daily to obey His will for you that day.

_____

_____

_____

_____

_____

_____

_____

Food in the Fast Lane

Sometimes I like to eat a good old-fashioned hamburger, French fries, and a milk shake from a local fast-food restaurant. I like the burger dressed with mustard, lettuce, tomatoes, red onions, and cheese. I cut mine in half, and I select the juiciest bites. I also choose my fries one at a time, adding a little salt, and then dip them into some ketchup. Sometimes it can take me two or three bites just to eat one French fry! Between each bite, I take a sip from my milk shake. Another fast-food favorite is pizza! There are many choices in selecting the perfect pizza—thick, thin, spiced, or stuffed crust—you choose. There is also a wide variety of toppings to add to your favorite crust, anything from plain cheese to "the works." I enjoy having a good pepperoni pizza and an order of breadsticks delivered from the local pizza place. The pizza arrives hot, and I can see the steam rise as soon as I open the lid. I look for the best piece with just the right amount of pepperoni. I choose a slice and eat it with a knife and fork—that way, not only do I eat smaller bites, but the cheese doesn't swing down and burn my chin! I cut a bite-size piece that has an equal amount of cheese and pepperoni, and I savor it thoroughly. Next, I take a breadstick, dip it in the accompanying sauce, and take a small bite. What a treat! I'm a double dipper, though, so usually no one wants to share the dipping sauce with me! But whatever the circumstance, I delight in my all-American fast food.

I actually find myself eating more crust or breadsticks than the cheese and meat. Jesus *is* the Bread of Life, and if you pay attention to your body, you, too, will find yourself craving plenty of bread!

eleven

ESTRANGED FROM GOD

In John 15:1–2, Jesus tells us, "I am the true vine, and my Father is the gardener. He cuts off every branch in me that bears no fruit, while every branch that does bear fruit he prunes so that it will be even more fruitful." Are you still sneaking away and bingeing on food? Or have you lost most of your weight and really gotten the basics of God's plan for eating, but you know God could do a little pruning on your eating? Wherever you are on this journey, you need to know that God is busy at work.

GOD PRUNES EVERY BRANCH THAT BEARS FRUIT

There have been a few times that I realized that areas of my life were not in total surrender to the desires of God, and the progression of my feelings was awful. The snipping of the pruning shears is uncomfortable and sometimes very painful. At first, I would search the Scripture or let God's Word fall open, but I would be looking at words that only stared me in the face. Usually, I had no idea of what my heart was actually doing or that I was in the wrong. I have to warn you that Satan is the accuser of the brethren, and he has tried many a time to make me mistakenly feel horrible—as if God were pruning, but it was really Satan tearing me down. During these times,

I would cry out to God to make sure that this pruning was from Him, and the Bible would open to the passage that says, "If anyone does attack you, it will not be my doing; whoever attacks you will surrender to you" (Isa. 54:15). You have to learn what is in your heart because Satan can falsely accuse you to get you to give up this incredible journey to God.

But in those times that I was truly convicted, I would repent—sincerely and fearfully repent. Later, I would turn to Scripture that says,

> "For a brief moment I abandoned you,
>   but with deep compassion I will bring you back.
> In a surge of anger
>   I hid my face from you for a moment,
> but with everlasting kindness
>   I will have compassion on you,"
>   says the LORD your Redeemer. (Isa. 54:7–8)

HE CUTS OFF EVERY BRANCH THAT BEARS NO FRUIT

A branch happens to be a part of the plant getting the sap. We are the branches getting the sap from Jesus Christ, the True Vine. Someone can be a branch springing up in Christ, but like the plant in the second soil in the parable of the four soils, it will die if it does not take root (Luke 8:6). People don't really believe that God cuts off branches that do not produce the fruit of repentance and a changed life.

Many times we believe we are abiding in Him, but we actually do not have a clue that we are a branch that is fruitless. God is an active Gardener. We must believe that. There are times when we have one foot in the temple while our backs are toward God—or we are a branch that is slowly losing the sap of Jesus Christ. We are experiencing less joy and peace because we don't produce fruit in keeping with repentance (Matt. 3:8). We seem to have less mercy for our spouses and coworkers, and we are not even patient with our pets.

What self-control we did have with eating has disappeared, and we do not know what is wrong. When we do not abide in Jesus Christ, we will not bear fruit; therefore, we must understand the responsibility of abiding.

True repentance means a *change of mind* brought about by *godly sorrow* that leads to a *change of life* (2 Cor. 7:10). Repentance is the major foundation of bearing any fruit. When you repent, the spirit of Jesus can come into your life. The fruit of the spirit of Jesus is "love, joy, peace, patience, kindness, goodness, faithfulness, gentleness and self-control," and it is manifested in many ways (Gal. 5:22–23). You need to have them all—not just one or two. Even pagans can have one or two of these without having the spirit of Christ. But Galatians 5:16–17a, 24 says, "So I say, live by the Spirit, and you will not gratify the desires of the sinful nature. For the sinful nature desires what is contrary to the Spirit, and the Spirit what is contrary to the sinful nature. . . . Those who belong to Christ Jesus [abide in Christ] have crucified the sinful nature with its passions and desires."

If you continue to bear no fruit, then you are cut off from Jesus Christ. But if you do bear fruit, you will go through some painful pruning from time to time so that you will bear even more fruit. I have been there. God has shaken me up several times so that I can see what I am doing wrong. He has always been a gentleman about it, but a couple of times, it was frightening. I have experienced being out of favor with God, and it is awful. I never want to go there knowingly. I do make mistakes. I have felt like a "Peter" and wept, and I have felt like a "Paul" when I have realized that I was hurting the cause of Christ but had no idea I was doing it. The Apostle Paul was zealous for God, and before his conversion he thought he was pleasing God by killing, imprisoning, and mistreating the "heretical" Christians. Paul had no idea that he was hurting Jesus—until he was knocked off his feet by a voice from heaven and a light that blinded him for three days. He was then baptized into the total following of Jesus Christ. At that time, it was understood that to be *baptized* meant to be totally indoctrinated, surrounded by, and immersed into the teachings. So to abide by or be baptized into Jesus Christ is to surround yourself with the heart and life-behavior of Jesus, who followed the will of the Father—not just on one day, but daily. Jesus took His will and set it on its knees before God the Father every day! The Apostle Paul repented, never to return to his old ways.

You see, God is a Redeemer. His defining characteristic is that He puts things back together more than He takes them apart.

You see, God is a Redeemer. His defining characteristic is that He puts things back together more than He takes them apart. Second Samuel 14:14b says, "But God does not take away life; instead, he devises ways so that a banished person may not remain estranged from him." The Bible describes the woman who said those words to King David as a "wise woman." This is a beautiful description of God and gives me great hope that a banished person may not remain estranged from Him!

WHAT HAPPENS WHEN A CHILD OF GOD IS CAUGHT IN A SIN

How does God handle someone who has been in love with Him and then he finds himself caught up in a sin? He didn't plan this. It wasn't his bent—but here he is with his back turned away from the Father and his heart loving someone or something else. I was curious about what happened to King David when he did this, and I read the whole account of King David and his sin in 2 Samuel 12 to learn how God handled this "man after his own heart." God did not prevent David from giving in to the sin of lusting after another woman, sleeping with her, and arranging her husband's death. However, I am sure our God provided a way of escape from David's temptation, yet David did not look for it. First Corinthians 10:13–14 says, "No temptation has seized you except what is common to man. And God is faithful; he will not let you be tempted beyond what you can bear. But when you are tempted, he will also provide a way out so that you can stand up under it. Therefore, my dear friends, flee from idolatry." David was so determined to have his way that he missed the way of escape.

Once David had committed the sin, he wasn't really aware that he had done something wrong. The Lord had an interesting way of waking David up. Listen to the following story from 2 Samuel:

> The LORD sent Nathan to David. When he came to him, he said, "There were two men in a certain town, one rich and the other poor. The rich man had a very large number of sheep and cattle, but the poor man had nothing except one little ewe lamb he had bought. He raised it, and it grew up with him and his children. It shared his food, drank from his cup and even slept in his arms. It was like a daughter to him. Now a traveler came to the rich man, but the rich man refrained from taking one of his own sheep or cattle to prepare a meal for the traveler who had come to him. Instead, he took the ewe lamb that belonged to the poor man and prepared it for the one who had come to him." (12:1–4)

After hearing the story, King David burned with anger and gave his own judgment. He said, "'As surely as the LORD lives, the man who did this deserves to die! He must pay for that lamb four times over, because he did such a thing and had no pity.' Then Nathan said to David, 'You are the man!'" (2 Sam. 5b–7a).

I bet David's heart died inside when he heard "You are the man!" He realized that he deserved to die. My guess is that some of the time, when you are mad at someone for doing something to you, it is God showing you what you are doing to Him. God is saying, "You are the man or woman—in sin." If my children are not being respectful, or if an employee has not listened to what I wanted but thought she was pleasing me by going her own way at times, I know that God is saying to me, "See—now how does that feel?" After feeling what God feels, I no longer want to treat God that way anymore. I want to be still and find out what He wants instead of pushing ahead on my own. My downfalls affect how I deal with people. Believe me, I show mercy to my children and my employees, for I need all the mercy from God that I can get.

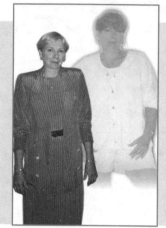

One morning as I knelt near my window to pray, I began recounting to God my 49 years of seemingly endless transgressions. One by one, as the tears poured out of me and I became sickened by the repugnance of my offenses, I offered God my true repentance and my heart. When I finally rose to my feet, it was startling how differently I saw things. Looking out that window during the past 17 years, I'd watched the trees grow and change with the seasons. This time my eyes drifted over the treetops to that old "t-shaped" utility pole on the hill. It now came into focus as a cross in my sights. Standing there, I reflected how God has helped me lose 34 pounds of accumulated burdens. I know I've just begun my journey . . . this time in the right direction.
Paulette Stover—Franklin, TN

Paulette Stover dropped 34 pounds in weight, and a lifetime of burdens.

What happened to King David when he realized that he had hurt God? What happened to Peter, the disciple of Christ, who denied Him three times? Well, they were disciplined by God, and yet they enjoyed until death a renewed relationship with God. God is the God of second chances. His mercies are new every morning if your heart is truly trying. God arranged for severe consequences for King David's sin: David lost two beloved children—a son he had with Bathsheba, and another son, Absalom. But later, after David's repentance, God blessed King David with another beloved son—Solomon—who rose up and ruled over the kingdom and was loved by God. I can vouch that His love is merciful and far-reaching.

As for the Apostle Peter, the pain of realizing he had hurt God (Luke 22:60–62) was enough for him. His relationship with Jesus was restored. In fact, Jesus promised to give Peter the keys to the kingdom, and Peter went on to speak powerfully and boldly for Jesus the rest of his living days, sharing sweet communion with the Father. Peter had such power that Acts 5:15 tells us that people longed to just walk in his shadow in hopes of being healed!

The common denominator of these men is that they sinned, were stricken to the heart, and then repented before God—that is, genuinely turned, never to return to the same sin. And finally, they lived even more powerfully for the Father (2 Cor. 7:10–11).

The point is that God knows the heart and the thoughts of man, and He disciplines those whom He loves. The Bible says,

> *Blessed is the man you discipline, O LORD;*
> *the man you teach from your law;*
> *you grant him relief from days of trouble,*
> *till a pit is dug for the wicked.*
> *For the LORD will not reject his people;*
> *he will never forsake his inheritance. . . .*
> *When I said, "My foot is slipping,"*
> *your love, O LORD, supported me.*
> *When anxiety was great within me,*
> *your consolation brought joy to my soul.*
> (Ps. 94:12–14, 18–19)

The Apostle Paul got up after the three days of blindness and went out, directly preaching the gospel of Jesus Christ within days after hearing the voice from heaven. If I had been Paul, I am pretty sure that I would have just passed out from fear.

When I find out that I have done something wrong before God, I also have a tendency to completely want to quit. I am afraid, embarrassed, and ashamed, and I argue that God needs only the best. I want to tell God, "Get away from me—I am a sinner." I suppose this is a very pouty, self-focused response to the disciplining of God. Once I said that to God, and the Bible fell open to Peter saying those very words. Look at Jesus' response:

When he had finished speaking, he said to Simon, "Put out into deep water, and let down the nets for a catch." Simon answered, "Master, we've worked hard all night and haven't caught anything. But because you say so, I will let down the nets." When they had done so, they caught such a large number of fish that their nets began to break. So they signaled their partners in the other boat to come and help them, and they came and filled both boats so full that they began to sink. When Simon Peter saw this, he fell at Jesus' knees and said, "Go away from me, Lord; I am a sinful man!" . . . Then Jesus said to Simon, "Don't be afraid; from now on you will catch men." So they pulled their boats up on shore, left everything and followed him. (Luke 5:4–8, 10b–11)

The comforting thought I got from this was not to be afraid. I had read this passage before, but never had I seen this response from Peter until I had felt the very same way.

The key to the heart of the Father is repentance. It is not to dwell on the things that you have done wrong, but to dwell on what God wants you to do and to become from this day on. This passage in Ezekiel 18:21–23 is direct:

But if a wicked man turns away from all the sins he has committed and keeps all my decrees and does what is just and right, he will surely live; he will not die. None of the offenses he has committed will be remembered against him. Because of the righteous things he has done, he will live. Do I take any pleasure in the death of the wicked? declares the Sovereign LORD. Rather, am I not pleased when they turn from their ways and live?

And Jesus' words are comforting. Look at His parable in Luke 15:4–7:

Suppose one of you has a hundred sheep and loses one of them. Does he not leave the ninety-nine in the open country and go after the lost sheep until he finds it? And when he finds it, he joyfully puts it on his shoulders and goes home. Then he calls his friends and neighbors together and says, "Rejoice with me; I have found my lost sheep." I tell you that in the same way there will be more rejoicing in heaven over one sinner who repents than over ninety-nine righteous persons who do not need to repent.

And in Jesus' parable of the lost coin He says, "In the same way, I tell you, there is rejoicing in the presence of the angels of God over one sinner who repents" (Luke 15:10).

First of all, I would like to point out that there are people on the journey who do not need to repent. That is encouraging to know. But we need to hear that the shepherd "joyfully puts the sheep on his shoulders and goes home"! I want you to know that there are heavenly get-togethers and rejoicing in heaven when just one lost sheep returns and repents. You may be on the Father's shoulders if you have laid down your idol.

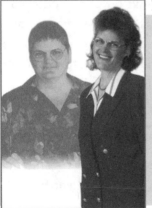

God had been to me a kind of magic guru in the sky. I pictured Him as the ultimate storehouse where I could go to get my every need met. But I never asked God what He wanted from me. I didn't consider that I needed to love Him first. Through Weigh Down†, God has drastically changed my life. He has melted 85 pounds off my body, and today I take no antidepressants! Every time I humble myself before God, confess my sins, and ask Him for the grace to live according to His will, He allows me to soar above food, anger, pride, arrogance, depression, or overindulgence of any type. I just want to share this message with anyone I meet. Repentance is the key to love and joy.
Theresa Giffin—Fall Creek, OR

Theresa Giffin found that when she gave herself to God, He filled her life with victory.

NOTE THE KINDNESS AND SEVERITY OF GOD

You cannot be "lost" and "at home" at the same time. When you turn from your old ways, God is very *pleased*—He's not mad at you. I believe that we sometimes still have to bear the consequences of our sin, as did King David. But God is pleased that we are sick of going against His will and that we now want to do things His way.

I believe that we all need to be careful that we are pleasing God, and I do not believe that we can box God up and say that He is always going to respond a certain way. He is sovereign and can do whatever He wants—that is why the Scripture warns us for good reason to "work out your salvation with fear and trembling" (Phil. 2:12b). Other Scripture warns us to note then the kindness and sternness of God: "Consider therefore the kindness and sternness of God: sternness to those who fell, but kindness to you, provided that you continue in his kindness. Otherwise, you also will be cut off" (Rom. 11:22). The King James Version says, "Behold therefore the goodness and *severity*." And look at the phrase "provided that you continue"—the *response* (ability) is ours.

Some personalities note God's kindness. Others note His sternness or severity and live each day consumed with fear of God's punishment. But the writer of Philippians wanted us to be balanced and realistic. We are made in God's image—and God's response is not so very different from our response to our own wayward children or to others when they hurt us. If you have a child who continually misrepresents your moral character, embarrasses you, and expects *you* to take care of his financial consequences—such as an illegitimate child—what do you feel like doing when he has not repented? What if he continually (for years) brings home larger and larger gambling debts and more illegitimate children? Now you can identify with God, the Gardener who cuts off branches.

When I feel as if I am out of step with God and I have taken advantage of His good nature and long-suffering, I do whatever it takes until I feel His peace and love again. I am on my knees and awake in the night to be in His Word. I am looking for signs and looking for His opinion of me. I don't assume that I will not bear any consequences—but I do usually beg God not to punish me. When I do feel consequences, I thank Him for His disciplining hand, and I humbly go on my way trying to please Him with every action and thought. The end result of it all? I am closer to God and understand Him better. This pruning from God is worth it all. His mercies are wonderful . . . but are not to be taken advantage of. Every time I have felt God showing me where I have gone against His will, I have repented immediately. It hurts to know that I have disappointed God. I am sure it would hurt even more if I were to delay repentance, ignoring His signs and His pruning.

Look at this passage that sums up the two responses to the Father's disciplining: "My son, do not make light of the Lord's discipline, and do not lose heart when he rebukes you" (Heb. 12:5b). Again, one person makes light of and has no respect for God's discipline. He doesn't take seriously the fact that the Father really does get mad. The person who thinks this way is more likely to repeat the offensive behavior. This is the child who has taken repeated trips to the principal's office and is not afraid of the fussing or the paddling from the coach. This is the person who has committed repeated affairs or is unwilling to let go of the food or drug or pilfering. When you get this far, to the point that you cannot be disciplined, then you are in trouble. Proverbs says much about the fool who rejects discipline, for example, "He who scorns instruction will pay for it, but he who respects a command is rewarded" (Prov. 13:13).

On the other extreme, there are those who lose heart. I personally fall in that category more than the other. The worry that I have displeased God almost paralyzes me—not literally, but mentally and spiritually. If I think that God is angry with me, it affects my work and my ability to make decisions. I know that this extreme can be a bother to the Lord. I know when my own children have lost heart, and so to cheer them up I try hard to input the perspective of the disciplining I am doing. It is hard to cheer the depressed. But in Genesis 4:6–7a, God said clearly to Cain when he did wrong, "Why are you angry? Why is your face downcast? If you do what is right, will you not be accepted?" Do you see how simple it is? If you do what is right, you will get the acceptance back that you are looking for! I love this God of ours! First John 3:7–8a states, "Do not let anyone lead you astray. He who does what is right is righteous, just as he is righteous. He who does what is sinful is of the devil."

So who does He accept as a son, as an offspring? Anyone who emulates Jesus Christ and abides in the True Vine. Anyone who continues in sin is of the devil and has not been born of God. "No one who lives in him keeps on sinning. No one who continues to sin has either seen him or known him. . . . No one who is born of God will continue to sin . . . he cannot go on sinning, because he has been born of God" (1 John 3:6, 9).

Let's continue with the passage from Hebrews 12:

Endure hardship as discipline; God is treating you as sons. For what son is not disciplined by his father? If you are not disciplined (and everyone undergoes discipline), then you are illegitimate children and not true sons. Moreover, we have all had human fathers who disciplined us and we respected them for it. How much more should we submit to the Father of our spirits and live! Our fathers disciplined us for a little while as they thought best; but God disciplines us for our good, that we may share in his holiness. No discipline seems pleasant at the time, but painful. Later on, however, it produces a harvest of righteousness and peace for those who have been trained by it. Therefore, strengthen your feeble arms and weak knees. (vv. 7–12)

We make mistakes with our hearts' choices, but we are to use the mistakes to turn around and get it right. In our weakness, we see God's strengths: caring patience, tender concern, captivating love, and perfect justice. You learn about yourself and the personality of God. Endure hardship because God is treating you as a son. If you are abiding in the True Vine, then you are a legitimate branch—a child of the sovereign God of the universe—and He loves you.

Children who continue in sin are the same as the prodigal son. The prodigal son took his entire inheritance, expecting never to return home or to the father. He committed many sins and squandered his body and his money with no fear and with seemingly no cares. He never even gave God a second look—until he was spent. No food, no friends, no home, and no job to speak of. He had gone past the pleasure of sin to the point that the sin had broken him financially, relationally and spiritually. Can you identify with this? Have you committed the same sin again and again until you hate your life and situation and just want to die? Well, don't do that. The prodigal son at least had enough sense to humbly go back to the father. And the father had been coming out every day, looking from afar, in eager expectation for his child to return home. God is looking for you every day to start that trip home. He is not going to dwell on the past. You are a child of the King and an object worth waiting for. He is going to put a beautiful robe on you to hide your tattered clothes from the past, so that no one will know how low you have been. He is going to feed you the choicest physical foods and spiritual foods so that you can grow up quickly in a relationship with Him again. You do not have to stay in the pigpen, my friend. This is a very personable God. He wrote the story and told it through His only Son, Jesus Christ. Go home and never take your inheritance—or your right to love—away from God's house again!

CONCLUSION

God is a Redeemer. His defining characteristic is that He puts things back together more than He takes them apart. Second Samuel 14:14b says, "But God does not take away life; instead, he devises ways so that a banished person may not remain estranged from him."

We've defined God's personality a lot. Make sure you understand that your response is most important. In my experience and in my opinion, it is best to work out this relationship with God with "fear and trembling." Show some respect. I would investigate as a detective does in a mystery. I would quarry like someone looking for gold. I would tunnel like a prisoner trying to dig his way out of prison. In the movie *The Shawshank Redemption,* a man was convicted of a crime and jailed for life. He spent twenty years digging with a tiny tool, tunneling his way outside. His tunnel was hidden behind a poster on the wall, and his tiny hammer was hidden in a carved-out area in his Bible. He dug every day and lost sleep every night as he was determined to get beyond the wall. Finally, he broke through the wall and climbed free, and his first action was to raise his arms to the sky—he was free after twenty years of digging! Twenty years! We spend just one hour publicly announcing to all that we want to invite Jesus into our hearts and oftentimes expect that to be all it takes. Examine the Scriptures, stay in the Word, and study the life of Jesus. We must chisel away through the rocky pieces of our hearts, even if it takes twenty years to find the freedom to love God with our whole hearts. Then once you have escaped the prison, stay far away from it.

How important is it to get in good with the greatest, most intelligent, purest, most powerful God of the universe? Who can live without answered prayers and comfort? Who can live without the sunshine of His face? Let's encourage one another to never do anything that would make us estranged from God and to sell everything and risk all to abide in Jesus Christ.

Getting in good with God is about repentance. We must learn that repentance—turning—is foundational to becoming a Christian. When you repent, your eyes are opened and you can see the truth. Second Corinthians 4:14–16 and 2 Timothy 2:25–26 back up this repentance-wisdom connection. Repent and live; repent and learn. This is the way back to God (James 4:4–10).

What You Can Do Today

~ *Go where God is leading you in Scripture.*

~ *Think about how you react to God's pruning in your life.* Remember that only the plants that are properly tended, cared for, and pruned back can continue to bear fruit, while the ones that are allowed to grow wild will grow out of control and will not bear any fruit at all. Instead of becoming angry at God or feeling sorry for yourself, recognize His loving concern and bow in humility before Him.

~ *Submit to His power and authority.* Do you lose heart when you feel discipline from God? Starting today, when you feel God's guiding hand pruning you, seek Him with an eagerness to repent and be the pure-hearted person He wants you to be. Don't lose heart—rejoice, for God is pruning you to bear even more fruit!

~ *When God reveals a sin in your life, take responsibility for it, repent, and live in pure devotion for God!* When King David realized his sin, he repented and accepted the consequences God brought upon him. The last time you were confronted with sin in your life, did you immediately admit your sin, repent, and accept the consequences before the Lord, or did you search for excuses, blame everyone else, and beg God to let you get by with it?

_____

_____

_____

_____

_____

_____

_____

Sports Games, TV, and Food

This is a great opportunity to take inventory of all the foods available so that you can select exactly what you want to eat when you are hungry. For example, when I attend a sporting event, I like to scan the menu at the concession stand *and* take note of the food vendors walking the aisles. I like to wait until I am good and hungry. That way, I can choose exactly what I want to eat. Sometimes I prefer a freshly baked pretzel covered in salt crystals from the concession stand or a corn dog smothered with tangy mustard and a bag of chips from the food vendor. I make sure that I am fully aware of the available food choices before I make my decision. Another common scenario is gathering with family and friends to watch a favorite team play a game of football, baseball, or basketball. With every gathering there will always be food! Yes, the chips surround the bowls of salsa, onion dip, cheese dip, and ranch dressing dip. Not only that, but there are three kinds of chips! There are plenty of pretzels, cheese puffs, peanuts, submarine sandwiches, crackers and cheese, not to mention dessert. The dessert selection may include ice-cream sandwiches, nutty bars, or cake and ice cream. Once I see what the selections are, I make my choices about exactly what I want to eat before I actually begin eating. After all, I wouldn't want to get full before I discover that cake and ice cream are available! It is important to know the food choices available to you. That way, you can have your cake *and* eat it, too!

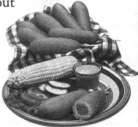

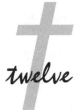

twelve

INNOCENT IN HIS SIGHT

We are told, "The weapons we fight with are not the weapons of the world. On the contrary, they have divine power to demolish strongholds. We demolish arguments and every pretension that sets itself up against the knowledge of God, and we take captive every thought to make it obedient to Christ" (2 Cor. 10:4–5).

In 1996, prisoners sentenced for drug offenses accounted for 60 percent of the inmates in federal prisons.[1] In a survey released in 1999, 78 million people, more than one-third of the American population, reported that they had used an illegal drug at least once in their lifetime, and 13.5 million said that they had used drugs at least once a month during the previous year.[2] The overuse of alcohol and tobacco is also growing. Excessive alcohol consumption causes more than 100,000 deaths each year in this country.[3] In 1998, 61 million Americans were habitual cigarette smokers.[4] Almost 13 million people are regular users of smokeless tobacco.[5]

The overuse of food seems to be the most acceptable overindulgence, not only in this country, but all over the world. More than one in three Americans are considered to be "obese,"[6] and if it continues to increase at the current rate, in a few years, one of every two people will be obese. Children account for most of the increase.

We Are Created with an Emptiness

Why do we have statistics like these? Well, God has created us to feel incomplete. Sometimes the feeling can be described as a deep loneliness. God wanted us to feel empty so that we would look for Him and perhaps find Him. In an effort to satisfy this feeling, mankind has mistakenly turned to alcohol, food, drugs, antidepressants, cigarettes, tobacco, or caffeine. This is a category that many have labeled as "substance abuse."

Only you know when you are depending on something other than God to help you make it through the day. There are legitimate physiological needs for some substances, such as when a juvenile-onset diabetic has to have insulin because the pancreas does not make it. Insulin is a gatekeeper, and it allows the food you eat to go into each cell. All the food you eat turns into glucose—the food for each cell in the body. If you do not have insulin, the glucose cannot get into the cells, and it just spills out in the urine, a telltale sign that you are very sick. Unless a diabetic injects insulin from an outside source at regular intervals in the day, death is inevitable. However, when I hear counselors compare this physiological need a diabetic has for insulin to the "need" a depressed person has for antidepressants—I just can't believe it. Life-giving drugs (such as insulin) cannot compare to the substances prescribed for moods that are not life threatening. Just a few decades ago, this country did not have access to drugs as we do today. How has generation after generation coped without all the drugs we take today or, in other words, handled depression tendencies?

When I refer to substance abuse, the substances I am talking about are the things that affect the brain and the central nervous system. These substances alter the mood of the person, or they are simply used for indulgence, such as the behavior found in overeating, binging-purging, or smoking. God created these chemicals and substances, and in and of themselves, they are not bad or evil or against the will of God. However, it is the dependence upon and worship of beer or liquor or drugs or antidepressants or the medicine cabinet that I am referring to. Take note of the following passages referring to wine:

He makes grass grow for the cattle, and plants for man to cultivate— bringing forth food from the earth: wine that gladdens the heart of man, oil to make his face shine, and bread that sustains his heart. (Ps. 104:14–15)

The Ephraimites will become like mighty men, and their hearts will be glad as with wine. Their children will see it and be joyful; their hearts will rejoice in the LORD. (Zech. 10:7)

Go, eat your food with gladness, and drink your wine with a joyful heart, for it is now that God favors what you do. (Eccl. 9:7)

All of these passages indicate that God knows full well why He created wine, and that its alcohol content was associated with cheering the heart of man.

Now as you enter the New Testament Scriptures, you see that Jesus' first miracle was turning water into wine (John 2:1–11). Why would Jesus use powers from God to create something that was against the will of God? Some people would have you believe that the wine referenced all over the Old and New Testaments was not intoxicating, but this is impossible when you read all of the wine passages in their context. In the Old Testament, Noah became drunk, and in the New Testament, the early Christians were chastised by the Apostle Paul because they became intoxicated at their own church services when partaking of the Lord's Supper (1 Cor. 11:20–22). Jesus commands us to drink wine and eat bread, and it was the last meal that He ate before His death (1 Cor. 11:23–26). Why, I pray, would Jesus Christ confuse all of God's children everywhere by commanding us to drink wine and yet God would not have us drink wine? It's because it never crossed Jesus' mind—or anyone else's. Again, the Bible teaches us, "The Spirit clearly says that in later times, some will abandon the faith and follow deceiving spirits and things taught by demons . . . [ordering] them to abstain from certain foods" (1 Tim. 4:1–3). Indeed, this teaching has come centuries after Jesus.

Elders and deacons were urged to have a list of characteristics that made them above reproach, and it included "not given to drunkenness" and "not indulging in much wine" (1 Tim. 3:3, 8). Both references indicate that wine, as always, was intoxicating, and both refer to overindulgence. But neither reference indicates that they should not drink *any* wine. It is ironic to note that we now have new rules taught by the deceiving spirit that state that *no* wine should be consumed. If we followed that man-made rule, Jesus Himself could not be a deacon in many churches today.

The overall teaching from Genesis to Revelation is *moderation* and learning to enjoy what God has made. It makes you feel differently about God when you realize that He wants your heart to be joyful, and therefore He created wine. You will not be able to find one verse in the Bible that backs up that God does not want us to enjoy wine. Those who want to continue in this legalism reference Romans 14, which is a passage about causing your brother to stumble. This is possibly the most abused passage in the Bible. It is thrown around by people who want to manipulate their viewpoint. How easy it is to say, "Well, you can't do that because I might stumble." Please read the entire chapter. This chapter is referring to doing anything that looks as if you are worshiping another god. In Rome, at the time of Christ, people would sacrifice animals and cook the meat and eat it. That was how you indicated that you worshiped or adored that god. The only way to apply that verse to us today is for us not to ever appear as if we are bowing down to another god. *That* could lead your brother astray. For example, if it seemed that you were having an affair (bowing down to the god of lust), but you were not, and someone was concerned, you need to make sure that you avoid the appearance of evil. "Eating food sacrificed to idols" was actually okay in God's eyes because God knows your heart is in love with Him and He is your true God (1 Cor. 8:4–8). If it looks as if your heart is in love with another god or idol on this earth, then be careful to clear this up with your brother. Drinking a glass of wine is not in this category. If that were so, Jesus would not have partaken, and Paul, who wrote these New Testament passages, would not have encouraged Timothy to drink wine in 1 Timothy 5:23.

I am well aware that people abuse alcohol, and that many people have died in car accidents as a result of drunk drivers. But never would I tell married couples to abstain from sex because wicked people abuse it. Never would I suggest that people stop eating because many are binge eating at ten o'clock at night. Therefore, I would never tell anyone to abstain from alcohol because some have mishandled it. Making God and what He likes and dislikes known should be our heart's delight. Likewise, distorting God's opinion should be scary.

Of course, there are legitimate times to take the drugs that God has created for the world. Even the Apostle Paul urged Timothy to take alcohol for his stomach problems, telling him, "Stop drinking only water, and use a little wine because of your stomach and your frequent illnesses" (1 Tim. 5:23).

But the world has labeled these substances as evil—never realizing that the heart of man and his overindulgence and abuse and dependency are evil. Satan loves this mind-set because we never get to the root of the problem so that we can be set free. If you do not understand that it is the *heart*—not the world—that God calls to behave, you cannot understand God. You will be confused. You will have built your house on the sand, and great will be the fall.

Most of the medical community and counselors have concluded that there are

If you do not understand that it is the heart—not the world—that God calls to behave, you cannot understand God.

chemicals found in each of these substances—such as nicotine in the cigarette, alcohol in the wine, sugar in the food, and caffeine in the coffee—that have strong addictive power over human beings. Even though my stance is radical, I maintain that the overwhelming magnetic pull of these substances is not from chemicals found in the food, alcohol, or drugs, but that the overwhelming magnetic pull is from the craving of the feelings or sensations that these substances provide, which is a counterfeit feeling that should be filled with a relationship with God.

If substance abuse is your stronghold, please understand that this is not a disease and that it is not a physiological addiction that causes you to binge. Eating a simple carbohydrate like sugar or chocolate will not trigger an uncontrollable binge. When people take the first taste, they often do binge until the chocolate is all out of the house, or until the alcohol is depleted, or the cigarettes are gone, and so on and so forth—but I want you to consider these different precepts that I propose about why someone would binge on food or would not be able to stop drinking.

Yes, I believe that there is *some* physiological addiction for the crack, cocaine, acid, alcohol, or cigarettes. Yet I am sure that it is not the major reason someone has a hard time stopping the alcohol or drug or binge-purge cycles or thirty cups of coffee a day. I know this is a new concept, but reconsider for one moment—the body does the best it can to accommodate carbon monoxide from the cigarette or calories from the 10,000-calorie binge or chemicals from the mood-altering drugs. For example, with alcohol, the body compensates so well that it has to take in more and more alcohol to have the same mood-altering effect. When you took your first drink, it might have really intoxicated you— but now it takes much more. The body builds up more of the enzyme alcohol dehydrogenase in the liver, so that it breaks the alcohol down more quickly instead of letting it circulate in the bloodstream longer. The body is trying very hard to break down the alcohol so that you are not overly intoxicated. The body is trying to make you moderate, and

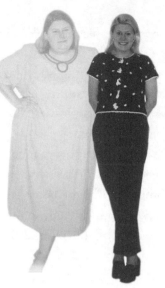

Before Weigh Down[†] and before having a close personal relationship with God, my biggest stronghold was negativity. I would walk through the forest and focus on the stump. Through Weigh Down[†], God has removed 156 pounds from my body, and I no longer take antidepressants or vitamins. There's no need for that. God fills it all. I feel so different now—I feel loved by Him, whereas before I felt hated by myself.
Kristen Hendrix
Midland, TX
Lost 156 lbs.

God has healed me from depression and thoughts of suicide, dropped 100 pounds off of me, changed me from a size 24 to a size 12, and given me a heart full of love for Him!
Debi Gades
Orlando, FL
Lost 100 lbs.

God used the Weigh Down[†] program and food to teach me how to let Him lead me and then translate that into a lifestyle. Because of this teaching and God's great mercy, I am happy to say that God has taken away my addiction to pornography and my homosexual desires. I am now filling my heart with His love instead of empty lies.
Anonymous

it does a good job—until it is overwhelmed with alcohol. Excessive alcohol consumption can cause cirrhosis of the liver.

I could go on and on with what we are doing to the body—the temple of God. Some damage is permanent, and the resulting accelerated aging begins to show up. In other words, people who have indulged often look older than their nonindulgent counterparts.

Withdrawal from drinking alcohol may cause delirium tremens in some alcoholics, which is a physiological reaction to the sudden deprivation of a substance the body is accustomed to. But the body actually welcomes this change. Just as the smoker's lungs want no more smoke and the overweight person's thighs want no more fat, the alcoholic's liver wants no more alcohol. It is not your body chemistry that makes you keep smoking or using drugs. It is not a physiological addiction, but a spiritual, or heart, addiction. The withdrawal is caused by separating the heart from its love for, or dependence upon, the substance. Since we were born to be attached to a superior complete Source, letting go of our other attachments may be emotionally difficult unless we transfer that dependence immediately to the one true Source, God Almighty. He is the complete Supplier of all things, and all needs, and all life.

I have seen people who have been addicted to drugs for thirty years who have experienced the transfer of this dependency to God, with no desire to go back. Once you have found God, you never want to return to the irritating side effects of prescription drugs or street drugs. You will be free to live a life of moderation, where you can take one drink, eat small amounts of chocolate, have an occasional cigar, or use drugs for acute needs that are short-lived, with no attachment. For people who are taking drugs, I warn you not to depend on them. Depend on God. After all, God makes the drug effective; God can take away the effect of that drug. He is the ultimate Creator and Doctor; He can do anything He wants with our bodies. So you had best be depending on Him and not making Him mad or jealous by having more faith in the medicine cabinet than in Him!

By the way, some people taking antidepressants will say, "Oh, they don't numb, and they aren't addictive." But then out of the other side of their mouths they will say, "I tried to stop taking them and 'crashed,'" or "I wound up in the hospital." What in the world are they taking that makes them wind up in the hospital if they stop taking it? Even someone drinking a glass of wine every night would not crash or wind up in the hospital if he stopped one weekend. What are you taking? Wake up and realize *Remember that you cannot just give an addiction up without replacing it with a close and loving relationship with God.* that drugs that affect your central nervous system must be stronger than you think. And please think twice before giving them to a child. Wouldn't Satan just love to keep most Christians numb to the leading of the Holy Spirit and numb to real joy? You must depend on God and ask Him into your heart.

THE GOD OF ALL COMFORT

If you decide that God is leading you to give up your substance abuse, remember that you cannot just give it up without replacing it with a close and loving relationship with God—no halfhearted efforts. If your usage is heavy, seek your doctor's recommendation for a reasonable progression for decreasing your dependence. Clinging to worthless idols causes depression. Remember Jonah 2:8: "Those who cling to worthless idols forfeit the grace that could be theirs." You need to give up the substance stronghold. Your heart will be happy as your body begins to recover, and the need for the drugs, alcohol, or food will diminish. Follow these steps:

1. Acknowledge that overindulgence is grabbing for a false comfort or god and trying to get a feeling when you want it instead of waiting on the true God to supply it.

2. Acknowledge that this substance abuse is a pit or a black hole that is hurting all aspects of your life.

3. Remember who is the God of all feelings and comfort. Get on your knees and repent that you have insulted God by trying to be your own god. Decide that you do not want to hold on to false comfort and these contrived sensations anymore. Tell God you think that His decisions for your feeling happy, or peaceful, or comforted are better than trying to create those feelings on your own.

    People have a perfectly normal need to be comforted, and only God can provide that comfort. He can do it with an encouraging word from a friend, a timely phone call, or an appropriate Scripture during your Bible reading. It says in 2 Corinthians 1:3–4, "Praise be to the God and Father of our Lord Jesus Christ, the Father of compassion and the God of all comfort, who comforts us in all our troubles, so that we can comfort those in any trouble with the comfort we ourselves have received from God." The other part of the healing process is to comfort others. Realize that you do not need the food, alcohol, cigarettes, caffeine, mood pills, or diet pills to fill you up. You are full of joy and unspeakable happiness! You are almost giddy with finding this give-and-take relationship with God and Jesus Christ.

4. If you want out, do not get sidetracked. Make sure you ask God to guide you to the truth. Too many groups or false counselors will teach the opposite of this Exodus teaching and will only leave you in confusion. Too many small group therapies subtly try to make you dependent on them first and then God. That is so wrong! Some groups will try to make you a lifelong member—that is not freedom for the captives that glorifies God. God's good news sets people free. When the whole truth is taught and applied, then you will see fruit! God can deliver you!

Be wary of those who try to provide you with miracle cures, absolute answers, or convenient excuses for your problems. Whatever the problem is, God is the answer. I have seen people overcome tremendous bondage to drugs, alcohol, and addictive substances when they persistently stayed on the right path.

Finally, remember that God knows what it is like to give up something He really wants. After all, He allowed His only Son to fall into the hands of evil. He watched the evildoers torture Jesus to death, emotionally and physically. Most of us don't endure suffering comparable to that of Christ. In fact, the Scripture tells us, "In your struggle against sin, you have not yet resisted to the point of shedding your blood" (Heb. 12:4). I know that this is difficult, but when you see that worshiping and depending on idols will separate you from the relationship and blessings of God, you will find a way out. Fight with all you have. Dig for God's approval and forgiveness as if you were digging your way out of a premature grave. Run away from the false sensations and prepare yourself for a small desert of having no great feelings or highs or sensations—a very dry time. Remember that you do not deserve to have anything that God does not give you. Wait for Him and you will eventually soar. You can't have the high of being pure-hearted before the Father and the high of substance abuse at the same time. The high that comes from pleasing God—doing it right, being innocent in His sight—is an unbelievably better feeling than the sensations derived from pills, alcohol, or cigarettes. Please make the only right choice—waiting on God to fill up your soul and mind and heart with an exhilarating acceptance from Him.

Look at what happened in Daniel 6. When Daniel was thrown into the lions' den, the good king was so upset that he did not drink or sleep the entire night. Then, the Bible says,

> *at the first light of dawn, the king got up and hurried to the lions'*
> *den. When he came near the den, he called to Daniel in an anguished*

Remember that God knows what it is like to give up something He really wants.

voice, "Daniel, servant of the living God, has your God, whom you
serve continually, been able to rescue you from the lions?" Daniel
answered, "O king, live forever! My God sent his angel, and he shut
the mouths of the lions. They have not hurt me, because I was found
innocent in his sight. *Nor have I ever done any wrong before you,*
O king." The king was overjoyed. (Dan. 6:19–23, emphasis added)

Daniel was found innocent in the sight of God Almighty. Oh, the
joy of fighting with all your heart, soul, mind, and strength to
remain pure and innocent in the eyes of God!

SEXUAL DESIRES

The next area I want to discuss is sexual sin. Sexual sin can take many
forms, one of which is pornography. In the U.S. the adult video business has grown dramatically from a $1.6 billion industry in 1992 to a
$3.9 billion industry with approximately 7,800 new adult titles
released in 1997.[7] In the same way, the adult magazine and adult television markets continue to grow.

Pornography, soap operas, sexually explicit television shows and
movies, and trashy novels are all readily available. Too much goes on
in America's offices as men and women lust after one another at
work. God knows the motives behind why you read certain articles
in a magazine or watch news about the stars. Are you wanting to
hear about an affair or a divorce? Are you planting and watering
seeds of a wandering lust in your own life? All of the sexual sins have
devastating results, often leading to divorce—but what is worse,
they can lead to a break in your eternal relationship with the Father.
First Corinthians 6:15–18 tells us,

Do you not know that your bodies are members of Christ himself?
Shall I then take the members of Christ and unite them with a pros-
titute? Never! Do you not know that he who unites himself with a

prostitute is one with her in body? For it is said, "The two will become one flesh." But he who unites himself with the Lord is one with him in spirit. Flee from sexual immorality. All other sins a man commits are outside his body, but he who sins sexually sins against his own body.

The U.S. Census Bureau reported in 1999 that there was one divorce for every two marriages in this country.[8] How can our hearts get so confused to believe that we were put on earth to satisfy our whims? Most people think the answer is to clean up the environment—but good luck! Satan is the ruler of this world, and he would just welcome you spending the rest of your life trying to campaign and clean up the world. But that was not what Jesus did—He came to get you focused on how to please the Father by cleaning up your own heart. He is the One who said in Matthew 5:27–30,

You have heard that it was said, "Do not commit adultery." But I tell you that anyone who looks at a woman lustfully has already committed adultery with her in her heart. If your right eye causes you to sin, gouge it out and throw it away. It is better for you to lose one part of your body than for your whole body to be thrown into hell. And if your right hand causes you to sin, cut it off and throw it away. It is better for you to lose one part of your body than for your whole body to go into hell.

Jesus taught us to master sin, not let it control us. He is a God of action verbs, and He has given us the ability to make the choice.

I can tell you that this category is a tough one because lust is truly inside the heart and it can be activated at any time. It is more available than food, drugs, or alcohol because the lustful person can turn on the TV, open a magazine, or just look around at work. God is harsher on this sin than others because it is blatant—body, soul, mind, and strength lusting after something other than Him. The mystery of marriage and the "oneness" that is obtained through marriage are very symbolic of our relationship with the Father. In marriage, your heart is to be purely and wholly devoted to the spouse God has given you.

Don't forget the Scripture that tells us to flee sexual temptation, and in Ephesians 5:3a, it says that "among you there must not be even a hint of sexual immorality." Not even a hint. This is going to take some conviction and refocusing in this country and in the body of Christ.

FLIRTING WITH FIRE

Well, how do you get out of the prison of sexual temptation? First of all, you must realize the danger of flirting with this fire. It usually starts off innocently enough, but you have to be careful. The righteous man, Job, said he made a covenant with his eyes not to even look lustfully at a girl, and he wished punishment upon himself if he even lurked at his neighbor's door (Job 31:1, 9–10). For someone with a food stronghold, it is dangerous to be playing around with lusting after or thinking about food. But playing around with a sexual stronghold is more dangerous. You must not play with this fire. Proverbs 6:28 compares adultery to walking on hot coals.

Sometimes sexual sin is not based on lust; instead, it is a behavior used for revenge on the spouse. How devastating—how cavalier! Do you think you can just get another wife or husband at the drop of a hat? God is the great Matchmaker, and He is Cupid, and He puts people together. If you play around with what He has given you, He may never bless you again. You must fear the consequences of this great lustful sin called adultery and realize that this is truly hurting the cause of Christ and the heavenly kingdom. It is insulting to God for us to continually want more than He has given. Satan loves to laugh at God as he throws the number of wandering and cheating hearts in the face of the Father, especially those who call themselves the church. The Greek word for "church" is *ekklesia,* and it means "the called out." The "called out" of the world have embraced the world, and it is embarrassing to the Father. Satan tells God, "They do not want You. Your children are not satisfied with what You give. See, I have been right all along! You do not deserve to be worshiped wholeheartedly. You (Your paternal nature, Your friendship, Your care) are not enough for man."

It is insulting to God for us to continually want more than He has given.

I do not want to give Satan any opportunity to laugh at the most wonderful heavenly Father and show contempt toward Him. It makes my blood boil when I think Satan is taunting God. When King David was greedy and wanted more, the prophet Nathan confronted him. David admitted his sin, and Nathan replied,

> *The LORD has taken away your sin. You are not going to die. But because by doing this you have made the enemies of the LORD show utter contempt, the son born to you will die.* (2 Sam. 12:13b–14)

Sin causes death; so God allowed death as a consequence of David's impulsive lust.

The dark world is full of enemies of the Lord, and the earth is full of enemies of the Lord. How could anyone not like God? I cannot comprehend it! Three in bed has *never* worked, just as God does not allow you and Him and an idol in the same relationship. The book of Proverbs states, "May your fountain be blessed, and may you rejoice in the wife [husband] of your youth. . . . May you ever be captivated by her [his] love" (5:18, 19b).

My advice, if you have this leaning or this temptation, is to go back and see what the cause is of your wandering eyes and heart. Some women think they are beautiful and have discovered that they can control men with this attraction—how sick to think that you are a god! If you are a woman leading a man the wrong way—how horrible to eternally know that you seduced another into a sin against the Father. This must be stopped. It is well known that men who are considered successful in life tend to have more affairs. The root problem is pride. If you are a successful man, and you are using your power to lead a woman the wrong way—how eternally horrible that you are trapping an otherwise innocent woman and defiling her. That was not why God gave you success—it was to glorify Him, not to defile the land and hurt innocent people.

If you are tempted because you think your spouse is unattractive, then you must accept what God has given you. Everyone has different gifts from the Lord. God has purposely given some more money than others, and some have better-looking spouses. Some have been given problem-free marriage situations but have difficult hurdles to rise above in their jobs. Life is not all equal. We are lucky to have even been given life and a chance to seek the Father and His grace-filled salvation! We should never want more than what God has decided to give. And to stop this craving, you had best get still before God and realize that He could uproot your harvest and take away the things that are important to you (Job 31:9–12).

There could be many reasons you play around with this fire, but the main point is to turn as you have never turned before and flee sexual temptations. Do whatever it takes to stop lusting on this earth, and turn your passion toward heaven. Think for one moment about being separated from the Source of love and the Source of life—the God of the universe. That would be unbearable. But being separated from your idol will not.

COUNT YOURSELF BLESSED

We have been given a shot at living forever with Jesus Christ and God the Father in a mansion above. Why throw this away? Why throw away establishing a peaceful life for your children? Why be greedy? It is a craving that will never be fulfilled. You risk throwing away the happiness sitting right in front of your eyes—a sweet family and children and possible grandchildren. The grass is *not* greener on the other side—that is one of the lies of Satan. Greed and jealousy are wrong. Life is not equal. We all have been given different positives and negatives or pros and cons so that we can glorify God from a castle or a mobile home. Life is totally fair in the sense that we all have an opportunity to love God with all the heart, soul, mind, and strength. If you have a beating heart, a soul, and a mind, then count yourself blessed. *Blessed.* Please concentrate on that thought. Equally concentrate on the fact that you do not deserve anything from God.

Recently, I had the pleasure of meeting Antony Thomas—a well-known writer, director, and producer who has won numerous awards, including a British Academy Award and an Emmy. He recently produced a documentary called *Fat,* in which he spent a week filming at The Weigh Down Workshop[†] office. This documentary has been aired in Europe, and it has had a great impact on opening more Weigh Down[†] classes in foreign countries.

Well, while Antony was in town, we viewed another documentary he had produced. The documentary was on twins, and one section had me practically spellbound. It was about Siamese twins who were connected physically at the head. Two totally separate people and personalities. One pursued voice lessons and the other enjoyed piano. Amazingly, they had separate brains, but they shared circulation of the brain's bloodstream. One twin was tall and the other very dwarfed. The larger one had learned how to walk bent over, with her

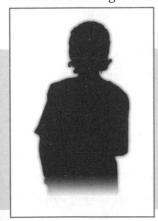

twin following in a specially made rolling high chair. Despite their disability, their

I remember that somehow pornography books became available to me as a child. My next-door neighbor had filthy videos, and I stumbled on them and was simply hooked. I knew it was wrong, but I didn't know how to escape. Through Weigh Down[†], God is teaching me what He expects from the body He has given me. I am to present my body as a living sacrifice, holy and acceptable to God, because it is my reasonable service. By the wonderful matchless grace of God, I am now free from the pornography and sexual sin of this world.
Anonymous

eyes beamed with joy. How could this be? Well, one reason is that they both had wisdom from God. Their parents never let them feel sorry for themselves or be selfish toward each other. They shared the hours each day by giving one another half of the day. In other words they could live only half a day doing what they wanted—and even that would be cumbersome. You could see that they got more joy from the giving than they did from the taking. They would never be able to have what most people had—but they were not asking God for more! They were happy and content with what they had. They would state clearly that they loved God, and they had the highest respect, love, and concern for one another. Well, I was glued to the whole documentary.[9] It verified my suspicions about life—we cannot feel sorry for ourselves and we cannot demand more from God, especially more pleasure. I believe the overwhelming reason that we have so many people hooked on soap operas, sitcoms, and lusting—even in the church building—is greed. We are showing God our hearts.

We are so overindulged in this country. We must think an awful lot of ourselves to go out and grab more pleasure from lust and sexual desires than what God has allotted. In Job 31:12a, Job called this "a fire that burns to Destruction" because there is no end to it. Ephesians 4:19 says: "Having lost all sensitivity, they have given themselves over to sensuality so as to indulge in every kind of impurity, with a continual lust for more." You will continue to want more and more, and you will eventually be given over to lust—but I promise you will *never* feel happy or fulfilled!

It verified my suspicions about life—we cannot feel sorry for ourselves and we cannot demand more from God, especially more pleasure.

So stop now and never go back. If you don't, you will ruin your life, your family, and your health. But what is worse—you will lose your relationship with the Father. Please listen. God's approval and what He decides to give you are all that matters! They will make you guilt-free, and peaceful, and joyful, with pure-hearted happiness so that you can look up at the heavens and smile.

I have quoted many times James 1:14–15, which says, "But each one is tempted when, by his own evil desire, he is dragged away and enticed. Then, after desire has conceived, it gives birth to sin; and sin, when it is full-grown, gives birth to death." Imagine the conception of evil in your heart. When a human baby is conceived, the fetus has a heartbeat after only twenty-four days. Imagine the heartbeat that your lust already has—don't give it any more time because it will give birth to sin or a misplaced devotion of your heart. Just as we read in James, once this monster in your heart is birthed, it will grow until it is fully grown, and when it is fully grown, it will give birth to death.

REDIRECTING THE LUST

How do you redirect this lust that has been filling up your day? Concentrate on the horrible consequences it brings. Living for your lust may be what gets you out of bed in the morning. It dictates your dress, your company, your TV programs, and your reading material. You like reading about it and talking about it. Well, you are flirting with death itself. Imagine yourself flirting with a corpse or a skeleton or the grim reaper. Read Proverbs again and again and again and memorize things like Proverbs 7:24–27:

> *Now then, my sons, listen to me; pay attention to what I say. Do not let your heart turn to her ways or stray into her paths. Many are the victims she has brought down; her slain are a mighty throng. Her house is a highway to the grave, leading down to the chambers of death.*

And from Proverbs 5:11–15, 18,

> *At the end of your life you will groan, when your flesh and body are spent. You will say, "How I hated discipline! How my heart spurned*

*correction! I would not obey my teachers or listen to my instructors. I
have come to the brink of utter ruin in the midst of the whole assembly." Drink water from your own cistern, running water from your
own well. . . . May your fountain be blessed, and may you rejoice in
the wife of your youth.*

And I love these verses in Proverbs 4:23, 25:

*Above all else, guard your heart, for it is the wellspring of life. . . . Let
your eyes look straight ahead, fix your gaze directly before you.*

If you do not repent, the families that you have hurt will always be
on your conscience before you. How awful to know it was all to satisfy a passion that would have died in a few days if you had not
fanned the flame and kept it going. You know how to put out a fire
at camp. Do the same spiritually—throw water on it—and cut off
the oxygen to this fire.

This is a heart issue. Jesus said that anyone who looks at a woman
lustfully has committed adultery in his heart. The same principle
applies to women, too. This teaching may seem very hard, but Jesus
was saying this for everyone's good. Who wants to be caught up in
an imaginary world? Instead, you could be transferring this lust to
your own husband or wife, and to passion for the heavenly Father
and His work and His kingdom. You would be investing something
rather than wasting it. What is more, you would get daily happies and
kisses from heaven. True love is something that will be returned.
Where your heart is, there is your treasure. On Judgment Day, if your
treasure is sex, it will not save you.

My friends, if you are facing this stronghold, then you are going to
have to dig your way out—back to the heart of the Father through
Jesus Christ, His glorious Son. Jesus has shown you how to die to your
will. Please do not give up hope that you can be set free from this spi-
derweb or this raging fire of longing in your heart. Proverbs 2:1–5 says,

My son, if you accept my words and store up my commands within you, turning your ear to wisdom and applying your heart to understanding, and if you call out for insight and cry aloud for understanding, and if you look for it as for silver and search for it as for hidden treasure, then you will understand the fear of the LORD and find the knowledge of God.

God will reward your efforts. It starts with something doable—staying in the Word and storing up God's commands in your heart. Crying out loud for insight and wisdom. Looking for the right path is like looking for silver or gold. Who cannot do this? Reading. Looking. Searching. Crying out loud. Applying your heart to what you are learning. *All* of us can do this. Victory is in sight!

Remember, you cannot clean up the environment around you. You have got to clean up your heart. But in the beginning, before your heart is strongly fixed on Jesus Christ, you must try to get away from anything in the past that has allowed you to indulge. I have known of people who quit their jobs because they were feeling strong sexual temptations. They were not sure where they would go and could not afford to miss a paycheck. But when God saw their love for Him and their determined commitment to Him, of course, He gave them an even better-paying job. I have also known of people to quit their profession because it was known to draw homosexuals, and again, God blessed them for their actions. So if possible, look for God's ways of escape and make a concentrated, full, heartfelt effort to avoid contact with people whom you know will give you a problem and lead you to temptation—even avoid eye contact if possible. Eye contact can be very powerful. That is why you must imagine yourself eye-to-eye with the Father. It will draw you in.

When you are tempted, physically remove yourself from the location and cry out to God. Try singing praises to Him. Satan hates that—and it will fill up your heart and end the longing. Always recognize the amazing ways of escape that show God's jealousy and loving desire to be close to you. Finally, imagine yourself side by side with Jesus Christ, your Brother, and God, your loving Father. God will give the victory, and you will soon have no battles to fight. You will live in peace with mankind and have no evil lust. There is life beyond the lust of the flesh, and the lust of the eye, and the pride of life. There is life fulfilling and life eternal with God. Wait on the Lord for feelings and fulfilled desires, for the Bible says, "The body is not meant for sexual immorality, but for the Lord, and the Lord for the body" (1 Cor. 6:13b).

FINANCIAL PROBLEMS

This category will touch on financial problems, love of money, deceit, greed, gambling, and more. Haggai 1:6b describes many people when it states, "You earn wages, only to put them in a purse with holes in it." In 1 Timothy 6:10a, Paul told us that "the love of money is a root of all kinds of evil." That root is interconnected to many of the strongholds that have been mentioned. If you really examine a lot of behavior and decisions made in life, it all boils down to craving money and wanting more and more of it. It boils down to lusting after money for its power because people think that it sets them free to do what they want. What they do not know is that God is in control and He could take away what they have—till they are living in a hut, having to go barefoot because they no longer own shoes.

If you are already in financial trouble, I am not going to give you a step-by-step process of how to cut up your credit cards and be debt-free. Just as I have taught that your being overweight is not the food's fault, financial trouble is not the credit card's fault. It is a matter of the heart. What I have witnessed again and again is that when you are sincerely broken and have come to the end of your "get-rich-quick" schemes and gambling ideas, then you are ready to depend upon God day by day, hour by hour. Financial seminars often suggest that you never buy anything unless you bargain or haggle with the seller (position buy), or that you buy only a house that has been repossessed by the bank in a foreclosure. These seminars are still putting the cleverness in your own hands, and this is not what I am recommending. Besides—have you considered that your "bargain" is possibly at someone else's expense? You do not have to "position buy" to get ahead.

What I recommend may seem strange to you, but it is real and it is a part of God's plan. First of all, you need to find out why you are in financial trouble. The answer is not that the bank gave you a high interest rate, or that your parents are greedy and won't help you out, or that your employer doesn't pay you enough. The real answer lies in your own heart—and the keys to being set free from this prison are in your hands. The reason you are in financial trouble is that you need to learn to seek His kingdom first and His righteousness. Then all these things will be added unto you.

This is deep and all-encompassing. Second, you need to learn all about greed and transfer your greed into a complete gesture of turning your hands palms up toward the Father, waiting on Him. Be content with what you have and imagine even less. You can be happy *with less.*

If you do this, you will see some amazing things happen to your material possessions and clothing and basic needs. And you will have almost inexplicable things happen to your bank account. You will know that God Almighty is doing what He promised He would do for the righteous. You will know that it is not through your own clever savings plans and savvy shopping ideas. You will realize without a doubt that you are to worry about God, His household, and His business first—and everything else will be added unto you. When you seek Him first, instead of caring more about your children and your home than about Him, He will bless you.

God is the God of behavior modification, and He will reward you when you are seeking Him and really caring about His kingdom before your own desires. Jesus gave us this principle in Matthew 19:29 when He stated, "Everyone who has left houses or brothers or sisters or father or mother or children or fields for my sake will receive a hundred times as much and will inherit eternal life." This is not only literal—this is also an attitude of the heart, and you can feel when His kingdom matters more to you than your own kingdom.

Once we were trying to sell our house, and I was praying, "God, why hasn't anyone bought my house yet? The last time we moved, You sold our house in two weeks." Well, I was on my knees, and in my mind I heard God say, "No one wants to buy My house." I started feeling His pain, for God has the *best* house, His kingdom is dynamic, and His house of truths is ingenious. That minute I told God I would be His real estate agent, and I would never worry about my own house again. I know God well enough to know He will take care of my house and my children if I take care of His house. He has given everything back. Let's go back to that passage from Haggai 1:

> Now this is what the LORD Almighty says: "Give careful thought to your ways. You have planted much, but have harvested little. You eat, but never have enough. You drink, but never have your fill. You put on clothes, but are not warm. You earn wages, only to put them in a purse with holes in it. . . . You expected much, but see, it turned out to be little. What you brought home, I blew away. Why?" declares the LORD Almighty. "Because of my house, which remains a ruin, while each of you is busy with his own house. Therefore, because of you the heavens have withheld their dew and the earth its crops. I called for a drought on the fields and the mountains, on the grain, the new wine, the oil and whatever the ground produces, on men and cattle, and on the labor of your hands." (vv. 5–6, 9–11)

I have discovered that since I sought His righteousness in my life and have been more zealous for His kingdom and His children than my own house, He has done more for me than I would have ever thought to do—and my children are so blessed by Him, more than I dreamed of for them.

GOD IS THE GIVER OF THINGS

Part of the problem we have had in this country is that we have taught everyone to grab all the gusto they can get and to take care of number one. We don't believe that there is a personal God who would multiply and expand what we have. We don't take God shopping with us because we're afraid that He might not like certain name-brand clothing. We don't believe that God would ever shop at all—much less for designer name brands. Well, I can tell you that God is the ultimate Shopper. I ask for His presence every time I shop, and I now have many treasures that I did not pay "treasure" prices for. God can take one dollar and give it the value of a million dollars—and on the other hand, He can take a million and turn it into a dollar. Proverbs 15:6 says, "The house of the righteous contains great treasure, but the income of the wicked brings them trouble."

God is the giver and we are to be content with what God gives. You are not to love God to get His money. You are to love God because you love His ideas and His ways, and you worship Him. The Apostle Paul said that

> godliness with contentment is great gain. For we brought nothing into the world, and we can take nothing out of it. But if we have food and clothing, we will be content with that. People who want to get rich fall into temptation and a trap and into many foolish and harmful desires that plunge men into ruin and destruction. For the love of money is a root of all kinds of evil. Some people, eager for money, have wandered from the faith and pierced themselves with many griefs. (1 Tim. 6:6–10)

Remember that for all strongholds—no matter what they are— pure feels better than all things. Empty feels better than full. Buying less at the store feels better than buying too much. "No indulgence" feels better than sexual lust. And having no money at all feels better than stolen money or contrived money. The truth feels better than the lie, and humility feels better than pride. When you overindulge, you feel sluggish—so energy feels better than lethargy. God can do better than a binge or an affair, and He can provide better than a million dollars. Are you tired of trying to fill yourself up? Then relax—unwind—surrender—give up and turn to God to fill your heart and provide for you. Learn the joy of letting God's approval and relationship be your everything in this desert of life. Drink from the only Water in the desert—Jesus Christ.

What You Can Do Today

Go where God is leading you in Scripture.

Examine your heart. Are you turning toward food or any other substance to fill your emptiness? Are you hoping God will just excuse your dependency on another substance? Stop asking God to excuse you. Instead, ask Him to *forgive* you as you honestly and wholeheartedly repent.

Make a list of any strongholds you might have in your life besides food. If you have died to your own will in favor of God's perfect will in the area of food, you know that you can do the same in these other areas! Recognize that just like excess food, these things will *never* give anything back to you or love you. Make the decision today to lay these strongholds down for good; they are worthless.

Realistically consider the consequences of having your particular stronghold. We all must endure the consequences of our actions. Besides damaging your relationship with God, being enslaved to a stronghold will damage many other things: your health, your family, your finances, and more. Turn it over to God, for He is the true Redeemer.

Turn your grabbing hands over, and wait patiently for whatever God decides to give you. God provides us with everything we need within His boundaries. Decide that you will not be greedy and that you *can* be happy with less. God will fill your heart with more than you can imagine!

_____

_____

_____

_____

A Special Occasion

Occasionally, my husband and I like to treat another couple to an evening at one of the finer restaurants in town. We enjoy the atmosphere, the dress, the candlelight, the soft music, the furnishings, even the fireplace burning—but especially our friends and each other. Remember to invite God into this special occasion! There may be many choices to make on the menu—a variety of appetizers, soups, salads, entrées, and desserts. I rarely start off with an appetizer. Instead, I may take a few spoonfuls of soup and concentrate on the luscious greens with just the right amount of vinaigrette salad dressing. Next, my entrée, duck à l'orange, arrives—a feat of the chef's creative genius. I then take a small bite of each item as I rate the foods on my plate. When I feel myself getting just the slightest bit full, I stop eating and push my plate slightly to the side. I want to save room for a few bites of their spectacular desserts! We usually ask for one or two desserts for the whole table to share. When the server comes to remove the plates, I ask for a carryout. At one of my favorite restaurants, the server brings your leftovers in foil that is artistically shaped. Who says it is improper to ask for a carryout from an exquisite restaurant? I always praise God, for He is the creative Genius and Artist behind each great surprise! We rarely eat at fancy restaurants, but anything in moderation is to be enjoyed. Keep in mind, though, that Proverbs 23:3 says, "Do not crave his [a ruler's] delicacies, for that food is deceptive."

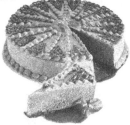

What is your motive for going to the restaurant? I pray it is not to lust after the food, but rather to glorify God, love others, and praise God for His genius, creativity, and boundless love.

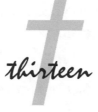

thirteen

THE REMNANT

And what was God's answer to him? "I have reserved for myself seven thousand who have not bowed the knee to Baal."

—Romans 11:4

Even if you have been going to church for years, I have found that most people rarely look at the overview of the Bible in terms of how God relates to man. There is definitely a clear pattern of how long God is willing to put up with rebellion and idol worship. If you still struggle with your overeating, then read this chapter. Knowing Bible history from Genesis to Revelation in regard to what God wants and what He expects will turn you from your binge eating forever.

In the Beginning

In the beginning God created the heavens and the earth. Now the earth was formless and empty, darkness was over the surface of the deep, and the Spirit of God was hovering over the waters. And God said, "Let there be light," and there was light. God saw that the light was good, and he separated the light from the darkness. God called the light "day," and the darkness he called "night." And there was evening, and there was morning—the first day. . . . And God said, "Let

the land produce living creatures according to their kinds: livestock,
creatures that move along the ground, and wild animals, each accord-
ing to its kind." And it was so. . . . And God saw that it was good. Then
God said, "Let us make man in our image, in our likeness, and let them
rule over the fish of the sea and the birds of the air, over the livestock,
over all the earth, and over all the creatures that move along the
ground." So God created man in his own image, in the image of God
he created him; male and female he created them. . . . God saw all that
he had made, and it was very good. (Gen. 1:1–5, 24, 25b–27, 31a)

Yes, God's creation *was* good—but after He created man, He said
it was *very* good. God was obviously pleased to have introduced
mankind, a creature made in His image who could respond in a loving relationship to its Creator. God was desiring to develop a loyal
people that He could call His own. Who of us on earth does not long
for loyal and loving friendships and devoted children?

THE FALL FROM PARADISE

It all started with Adam and Eve in Paradise. Eden was an incredible
environment for enjoying the artwork of God's hand, discovering all
the animals, trees, flowers, and brooks—everything that described
the genius of God's endless creativity and His boundless love.
However, Adam and Eve were not good candidates for returning a
pure friendship with God because they took advantage of His generosity. God gave them all but one thing, and yet they were greedy
and distrustful. You cannot have a relationship without trust.

Adam and Eve were the type who could be deceived into believing
false accusations from Satan concerning God—their superior. "You
will not surely die," the serpent said to the woman. "For God knows
that when you eat of it your eyes will be opened, and you will be like
God, knowing good and evil" (Gen. 3:4–5). God was such a loving
God that they were sure nothing would happen to them if they went

their own way—the masterpiece lie of Satan. With the first false accusation of this wonderful, generous Friend and "want-the-best-for-you" God, Adam and Eve did not hesitate to buy into the spirit of suspicion. They dived right in and showed this power-hungry God a thing or two! They would eat of the one tree in a world of freedom that they were told not to eat. They did not comprehend—even from seeing all of His creation—the personality of God, or they would have known that they would fall from Paradise. *Their* God didn't do things like that. How many times have I heard that one?

Personalities that are very loving, such as God's, are often taken advantage of. Why weren't Adam and Eve more interested in finding out what God wanted? Why would they buy into Satan's first lie that said God was not letting them in on the Tree of Life because God was power-hungry and did not want them to have more power? Their greed for more blinded them.

They dived right in and showed this power-hungry God a thing or two! They would eat of the one tree in a world of freedom that they were told not to eat.

Adam and Eve did not believe the warning that they would surely die. Why don't people believe in finality? Why do people feel that they are going to live forever? Why do they ignore death and lost relationships? Have you ever seen two-year-olds who want to squirm out of their fathers' arms and take off running into the traffic? Where is fear? Where is humility? God must see mankind as a world of two-year-olds darting here and there, thinking that we know what we are doing and we don't need a heavenly Father.

Instead of wiping out Adam and Eve, God graciously removed them from the ultimate blessings of Paradise and made them think about what they had done for the rest of their lives. Yes, God is loving, but that doesn't mean you can take advantage of that love. In a fallen world, Adam and Eve had to work harder, which taught them the attitude of appreciation—the quality necessary for an acceptable relationship.

Again, who of us on earth does not long for loyal and loving friendships and devoted children? And who of us does not know the pain of thinking that we have it, only to be let down? Oh, the pain that we have caused a God who deserves only the best time-honored appreciation and sincere love for what He has given. It is very unfair.

The Remnant

By the sixth chapter of Genesis, not long into the history of mankind, men began to increase in number, and the Bible tells us, "The LORD saw how great man's wickedness on earth had become" (6:5a). In fact, the Bible tells us that "every inclination of the thoughts of his [man's] heart was only evil all the time. . . . So the LORD said, 'I will wipe mankind, whom I have created, from the face of the earth—men and animals, and creatures that move along the ground, and birds of the air—for I am grieved that I have made them.' But Noah found favor in the eyes of the LORD" (Gen. 6:5b, 7–8).

Now the Bible tells us, "Noah was a righteous man, blameless among the people of his time, and he walked with God" (Gen. 6:9b). But since the earth was corrupt in God's sight and full of violence, God told Noah that He was going to put an end to all people—He was going to destroy both mankind and the earth. However, God planned to spare a remnant of eight people, so He told Noah to build an ark one and a half football fields long, almost a football field wide, and taller than a three-story building. Noah was to make a roof on it eighteen inches from the top. God told Noah to put a door in the side of the ark.

God told Noah that He was going to bring floodwaters on the earth to destroy all life under the heavens—that is, every creature that has the breath of life in it. God told him that everything on earth would perish. Genesis 6:18 says, "But I will establish my covenant with you, and you will enter the ark—you and your sons and your wife and your sons' wives with you." God told Noah that he would have to make room in the ark for at least two of all living creatures, male and female, to keep them alive with him. Noah was also to fill the ark up with food. "Noah did everything just as God commanded him" (Gen. 6:22).

It took one hundred years for Noah to build the ark, and during that time, the wicked people made fun of him. Just as people never believed that the *Titanic* was sinkable, the wicked never believed that the earth could flood. "Their" God, they said, would never do such a thing. What makes man think that God doesn't mean business? Or that God allows immortality? No, it is very clear that He has made us mortal. Our days are numbered, and our chances to respond to God's love are numbered. But the whispering voice of arrogance from Satan says, "You have time," and "You're immortal," and "There is no judgment."

Seven days before the floodgates would open, God commanded Noah, his three sons, and their wives to get on the ark. He told Noah he would be saved because God had found him righteous in this generation. God brought every kind of animal and every kind of creature that moves along the ground to Noah. He told Noah that it was going to rain for forty days and forty nights. Again the Bible tells us that Noah did all the Lord commanded him. Noah and his family and all the animals went inside this massive structure one and a half football fields long, and then the Lord shut them in. Noah and his family started to wait, listening for the evidence of rain. With each passing day, the sky grew darker and the clouds grew thicker.

The seventh day after Noah and his family entered the ark, the floodgates were about to open. The earth was rumbling. The wind was blowing, and the sky was darker than they had ever seen it. After generations of ignoring the signs from God, this generation, I am sure, ignored the purple sky and the rumbling earth and went on about their daily business.

You would like to think that this generation would have noticed seven days of clouds and thunder and turned to the Lord. You would hope that this generation would have noticed an ark (one and a half football fields long) sitting in the middle of nowhere. You would also think that people might start asking questions when the rumors went around about every kind of animal you could possibly think of lining up in Noah's backyard. But that is just like the wicked. They're blind and they're proud . . . of what, I don't know, because they just don't get it. Ignorance, stubbornness, and unrepentant hearts were left outside the ark. And the earth started to vibrate.

The springs of the great deep burst forth, and the floodgates of the heavens were opened. The "unfloodable earth"? Well, it began to swim with water. As the wicked were drowning, the righteous started to feel the wooden ark float. The door of salvation was sealed shut.

You might think that Noah would have had a bleeding heart for the people pounding on the side of the ark to get in, but you'll have to understand that Noah had been a preacher of righteousness, and that God's guiltless men are tormented in their blameless souls by the lawless deeds that they see day after day (2 Peter 2:5, 8). Besides, Noah knew God, which meant he knew the God who brings judgment. Noah did not have a problem with that, for he was righteous.

The "unfloodable earth" began to swim with water. As the wicked were drowning, the righteous started to feel the wooden ark float.

For forty days, the rain kept falling on the earth. As the waters increased, they lifted the ark high above the earth. As the winds tossed the ark to and fro, and the lightning flashed and thunder crashed, God kept the righteous safe in the ark. The waters rose to the point that all the high mountains under the entire heavens were covered to a depth of more than twenty feet.

Finally, at the end of forty long days of thunderous rain, the floodgates closed and the rain stopped falling from the sky. Every living thing that moved on the earth had perished: birds, livestock, wild animals—*all* the creatures that swarmed over the earth, including mankind. Everything on the dry land that had the breath of life in its nostrils had died. Only Noah and those with him on the ark were left.

All they could hear now was the sound of the wind and water lapping on the side of the boat.

God was starting over with good seed, hoping once again that He could have a people who would truly love Him with all their hearts, their souls, their minds, and their strength. What good seed to start with! This patriarch would pass down a faith that would work on an ark for one hundred years without any evidence or proof that it would float.

The Desert Remnant

Adam and Eve did not suspect that God would kick them out of Paradise, and the wicked did not think that God would send a flood. Paradise was history. The wicked were no longer on the face of the earth. Finality, judgment, and death are realities of God's personality and God's kingdom. However, a remnant of believers were saved, and God started over, seeking an undefiled relationship with mankind.

Time passed and arrogance grew after Noah's death. In fact, God had to separate the pride of man by making different languages at the Tower of Babel, and He had to send fire from heaven to burn up the wickedness in Sodom and Gomorrah.

We are thankful that God found another man who was pure-hearted. Abraham would be willing to sacrifice his own son for the will of God. He understood fully and trusted in God completely. God gathered the offspring of Abraham and allowed them to experience slavery. He would later rescue them from the wicked slave master, Pharaoh. God hoped that His people would then be able to appreciate His leadership as a good Lord and Master.

Mankind has a hard time distinguishing good from evil. As Adam quickly fell for Satan's lie about God in the middle of Paradise, God's children rebelled against God's loving leadership in the desert under the cloud and fire. God was overly patient, but eventually, their disobedience led to death, and their bodies lined the desert (Heb. 3:17b).

Only a remnant of the next generation would cross over the Jordan to try again to establish a pure-hearted relationship with God. This new remnant, through Joshua, would cry out, "As for me and my household, we will serve the LORD"! (Josh. 24:15b). This remnant had seen God's wrath, and they rejoiced in the fear of the Lord.

It wasn't that these generations didn't believe there *was* a God—as the Bible says, even the demons believe and tremble. All of these people prayed to God, they were called God's children, and they held true to a few rules and laws. But as centuries passed by, even the spared generations would see more and more blood from the throats of unblemished goats, rams, bulls, and lambs because the majority of people would rather *sacrifice* than *obey*.

THE FALL OF JERUSALEM

The covenant of God and His protection were true and sure. He would always be the good Friend, Lover, Husband, Warrior, and King of the people—a history of more than one thousand years of preferential care. Jerusalem was "the city of God, the holy place where the Most High dwells" (Ps. 46:4b). The children of God over the next thousand years would believe—correctly—that God wanted to dwell in Zion, but also—incorrectly—that she would never fall. Psalm 132:13–14 says,

> For the LORD has chosen Zion,
>   he has desired it for his dwelling:
> "This is my resting place for ever and ever;
>   here I will sit enthroned, for I have desired it."

Unfortunately, no matter how much God showed that He had chosen these people to love, the people would not believe that God would cut them off until it was too late. Satan's masterpiece lie was handed down from generation to generation.

God cried out through the prophet Jeremiah, "What fault did your fathers find in me, that they strayed so far from me?" (Jer. 2:5b). God's vineyard was dried up and the fig trees were ruined. The bark was eaten by locusts until the branches were white (Joel 1:7, 12). God was asking, "What more could have been done for my vineyard than I have done for it? When I looked for good grapes, why did it yield only bad?" (Isa. 5:4).

This relationship with mankind was definitely one-sided. God had intended for history to be there as a warning. You would think that the history of man's fall in Paradise, the Flood, the Tower of Babel, Sodom and Gomorrah, and the dead bodies in the desert would be warning enough. While on the other hand, the original gift of Paradise, the salvation of Noah, the blessings for Abraham, and the Promised Land for Israel would be positive reinforcement enough to give God the repentant and pure-hearted response that this good God of the universe deserves.

God would always be the good Friend, Lover, Husband, Warrior, and King of the people—a history of more than one thousand years of preferential care. Jerusalem was "the city of God, the holy place where the Most High dwells" (Ps. 46:4b).

After repeatedly warning Jerusalem to repent from its unrequited love, God started predicting through the prophet Jeremiah that He would have to form a new covenant with Jerusalem. He would send a Savior because the outside forces of the law, with all its policemen, were not encouraging the inside of the heart to love and obey. God was ready to get rid of ritual and form; He was preparing to instigate Spirit and truth.

"The time is coming," declares the LORD, "when I will make a new covenant with the house of Israel and with the house of Judah. It will

not be like the covenant I made with their forefathers when I took them
by the hand to lead them out of Egypt, because they broke my covenant,
though I was a husband to them," declares the LORD. *"This is the*
covenant I will make with the house of Israel after that time," declares
the LORD. *"I will put my law in their minds and write it on their hearts.*
I will be their God, and they will be my people. . . . Because they will all
know me, from the least of them to the greatest." (Jer. 31:31–33, 34b)

God's hope was that Jerusalem would repent when it saw Jesus
face-to-face. But it was not to be. Before Jesus' death, He would look
out one more time over God's desired Jerusalem and weep, saying,

O Jerusalem, Jerusalem, you who kill the prophets and stone those
sent to you, how often I have longed to gather your children together,
as a hen gathers her chicks under her wings, but you were not will-
ing! Look, your house is left to you desolate. . . . If you, even you, had
only known on this day what would bring you peace—but now it is
hidden from your eyes. The days will come upon you when your ene-
mies will build an embankment against you and encircle you and hem
you in on every side. They will dash you to the ground, you and the
children within your walls. They will not leave one stone on another,
because you did not recognize the time of God's coming to you. (Luke
13:34–35a; 19:42–44, emphasis added)

Jerusalem was an incredible city, built of gleaming white marble,
the city of the Most High. But Jesus wept for it because He saw the
heart of Jerusalem, and He knew the judgment on an unresponsive
people. God was willing—but the people were not!

When Jesus came, it was God coming down to earth, begging us
to repent face-to-face.

Then Jesus began to denounce the cities in which most of his miracles
had been performed, because they did not repent. "Woe to you,

Korazin! Woe to you, Bethsaida! If the miracles that were performed in you had been performed in Tyre and Sidon, they would have repented long ago in sackcloth and ashes. But I tell you, it will be more bearable for Tyre and Sidon on the day of judgment than for you. And you, Capernaum, will you be lifted up to the skies? No, you will go down to the depths. If the miracles that were performed in you had been performed in Sodom, it would have remained to this day. But I tell you that it will be more bearable for Sodom on the day of judgment than for you." (Matt. 11:20–24)

The hearts of the chosen people had grown cold, and when God, through Jesus, was face-to-face with the people, even He could not talk them into repenting. When God on earth said judgment was coming, they just couldn't muster up a care! The religious leaders of the day would crucify the voice that confronted them, for they were living for the "here and now." Not even the Son of God could talk Jerusalem into being a fruitful vineyard for the Lord. From Paradise to Jerusalem, God's chosen bride had refused wholehearted devotion to Him. The people were totally confident that the God they served overlooked sin. Because of this attitude, Jerusalem's selected favor was drawing to a close as its people continued to snub the warnings of the prophets and the miracles of God.

> *The hearts of the chosen people had grown cold, and when God, through Jesus, was face-to-face with the people, even He could not talk them into repenting.*

Indeed, the prophets had given plenty of warning:

The word of the LORD came to me: "Son of man, this is what the Sovereign LORD says to the land of Israel: The end! The end has come upon the four corners of the land. The end is now upon you and I will unleash my anger against you. I will judge you according to your

*conduct and repay you for all your detestable practices. I will not
look on you with pity or spare you; I will surely repay you for your
conduct and the detestable practices among you. Then you will know
that I am the LORD. This is what the Sovereign LORD says: Disaster!
An unheard-of disaster is coming. The end has come! The end has
come! It has roused itself against you. It has come! Doom has come
upon you—you who dwell in the land. The time has come, the day is
near; there is panic, not joy, upon the mountains. I am about to pour
out my wrath on you and spend my anger against you. . . . I will not
look on you with pity or spare you."* (Ezek. 7:1–9a)

The true personality of God was always prophesied by the true
prophets but soft-sold by the false pastors of the day. God called
them "mute dogs" (Isa. 56:10), because they could not bark or warn
God's people of judgment. This is true today as well.

THE REMNANT AT PENTECOST: THE NEW JERUSALEM

Finally, God ended this exclusive relationship with Jerusalem and
decided to allow any willing to hear—even the Gentiles—to have a
chance at this wholehearted, fearful but loving relationship with Him.
From Paradise to the rescue from Egypt to the alluring desert (Hos. 2:14), God's chosen bride had refused Him, with the exception of a remnant of people through whom the Seed would come. Jerusalem's time as a favored city was history. Jesus with His miracles had exhausted any means to get to the heart of Jerusalem. By A.D. 70, as Jesus had predicted (Luke 21), the forces of the Roman emperor Titus broke through the walls of Jerusalem, looted and burned the temple, and carried off the spoils to

Rome. As prophesied, the Holy City was totally dismantled and over-come. Every synagogue in Palestine was burned to the ground. There were great famine and widespread torture.

A pattern had developed: God offers an opportunity to be a child in His kingdom, and then He pleads and warns—up to a point. Then finally, there are judgment, destruction, and annihilation. The Scripture is clear:

> *If only you had paid attention to my commands,*
> *your peace would have been like a river,*
> *your righteousness like the waves of the sea.*
> *Your descendants would have been like the sand,*
> *your children like its numberless grains;*
> *their name would never be cut off*
> *nor destroyed from before me.* (Isa. 48:18–19)

If only we would pay attention.

The Christians were not destroyed in the siege, because those who believed had been warned by Jesus to flee from the city when they saw it being surrounded by armies. In fact, Luke 21 says:

> *When you see Jerusalem being surrounded by armies, you will know that its desolation is near. Then let those who are in Judea flee to the mountains, let those in the city get out, and let those in the country not enter the city. For this is the time of punishment in fulfillment of all that has been written. How dreadful it will be in those days for pregnant women and nursing mothers! There will be great distress in the land and wrath against this people. They will fall by the sword and will be taken as prisoners to all the nations. Jerusalem will be trampled on by the Gentiles until the times of the Gentiles are fulfilled.* (vv. 20–24)

At this point in history, we all have to feel for God—for how embarrassing to be spurned again and again by those you have chosen, to the

point that you have to start over with a new remnant! But that's
exactly what God did; He started over with 120 believers on the day
of pentecost (Acts 1:15).

The early Christians were baptized into this teaching and way of
life. *Repentance* and *obedience* were foundational, fundamental, and
essential to the new covenant, just as they were to the old. The difference would be that through Jesus' sacrifice, your past sins would
be forgiven, not rolled forward; you would be called to set aside your
own spirit or will and replace it with the Holy Spirit and His will.
You would not continue in sin, and you would walk in the light from
now on. If you did sin or stumble, you would have an Advocate with
the Father through Jesus' blood, and upon your confession and repentance, Jesus' blood would wash you free from all sin. Another way
to say this is that if we stayed in the light and not darkness, we could
see the dirt—or sin—and repent by following the footsteps of Jesus
and embracing the cross; the blood from the cross "purifies us from
all sin" (1 John 1:7b). In addition, because of Jesus' sacrifice, God
would live in our hearts, and the spirit of Christ would enable us to
overcome the world (1 John 5:3–4).

The law had been an outside force encouraging us to behave, but
now the Holy Spirit of God inside us would cry out to the Creator,
"Abba, Father!"—enabling us to be slaves to righteousness and to die
to sin. With the old covenant, a priest would take an unblemished
animal and go into the Most Holy Place, a special room in the temple,
to sacrifice it for the sins of the people. With the new covenant,
when Jesus was crucified, the curtain of the Most Holy tore (Matt.
27:51), and God called each of us to be a priest (1 Peter 2:5). In other
words, each of us, through the sacrifice of Jesus Christ, could go
through the curtain and into the presence of the great I Am. This
was not just good news. This was *extraordinary* good news!

Whereas the temple was a physical structure, now the temple is
the body (1 Cor. 6:19). Where worship used to be in Jerusalem or on
the mountain, now you cannot say that the kingdom of God is here

or there (John 4:21–22). Jesus explained that the kingdom of God is within you (Luke 17:21), and He explained that now worship is to be in Spirit and in truth, twenty-four hours a day, seven days a week. Jesus founded the *ekklesia*—"the called out." But over the centuries, the translation has lost its meaning. We've translated "the called out" into the word *church,* which has come to mean a building rather than a heart that has repented from loving this world. Satan loves to play with words that will slowly take away your response and conviction. Jesus is the Rock upon which the church—or "the called out"— was founded. He taught the apostles, who later recorded this passage for the early converts:

> *As you come to him, the living Stone—rejected by men but chosen by God and precious to him—you also, like living stones, are being built into a spiritual house to be a holy priesthood, offering spiritual sacrifices acceptable to God through Jesus Christ. . . . But you are a chosen people, a royal priesthood, a holy nation, a people belonging to God, that you may declare the praises of him who called you out of darkness into his wonderful light.* (1 Peter 2:4–5, 9)

All the realities had faded into symbolism through Jesus Christ. They understood the spiritual house, where you would offer your body as a living sacrifice, and the spiritual sacrifices that were all going on inside the heart of man. Romans 12 states, "Therefore, I urge you, brothers, in view of God's mercy, to offer your bodies as living sacrifices, holy and pleasing to God—this is your spiritual act of worship. Do not conform any longer to the pattern of this world, but be transformed by the renewing of your mind. Then you will be able to test and approve what God's will is—his good, pleasing and perfect will" (vv. 1–2).

With the new covenant, when Jesus was crucified, the curtain of the Most Holy tore, and God called each of us to be a priest.

The True Church Lost Its Foundation

This renewing means that inside your heart and mind and soul, you are putting that food or stronghold on the altar and killing it. The early Christians understood the Scriptures that said you were called to be pure and holy because you are now the physical representative of the church—the called out—the temple of God. The first Christians correctly worshiped seven days a week in public places and from home to home. They grew in number and were unified because they didn't establish a kingdom on every corner under a different name. And there was only one church, with one set of elders or shepherds, per city—even when there were 1.5 million people in Rome and 650,000 in Corinth.[1]

They understood the spiritual house, where you would offer your body as a living sacrifice, and the spiritual sacrifices that were all going on inside the heart of man.

That was the new picture of the New Jerusalem, and God was going to walk among His people and be in His people. Now He could have this relationship that He had been longing for. It is frightening that through the centuries, this church, founded in the heart of man, has faded back from symbolism and into physical structures. For most worshipers, the church now means the building, and worship is back to one day a week. The holy priesthood is viewed as the few people up front every Sunday, and repentance is something we want the government, school system, and abortion clinics to do!

Hear me when I say that God is shaking us all up now as we begin the twenty-first century to help us to restore this true picture of the church. Recently, God did a mighty shaking inside me that has led me out of complacency and contentment with the way things are. He has opened up my eyes to see the current state of His church and to warn all of the judgment that we are now under. John 9:39 tells us, "Jesus said, 'For judgment I have come into this world, so that the blind will see and those who see will become blind.'" In other words, many will recognize this counterfeit religion, and many will not.

He is calling His church to unify. People can do that—buildings cannot. He is calling the "called out" to repentance, and He is calling all lambs to understand this holy priesthood—that they are to be pure and holy in this choice of devotion. Instead of relying on a few people in the front of the building to lead us in worship, He is calling for us to get the foundations right in our hearts—in this temple (the body)—and for us to grow up because God is judging the counterfeit church.

Paul wrote,

> By the grace God has given me, I laid a foundation as an expert builder, and someone else is building on it. But each one should be careful how he builds. For no one can lay any foundation other than the one already laid, which is Jesus Christ. . . . Don't you know that you yourselves are God's temple and that God's Spirit lives in you? If anyone destroys God's temple, God will destroy him; for God's temple is sacred, and you are that temple. (1 Cor. 3:10–11, 16–17)

This passage offers so much for the body of Christ today. Knowing that the church is not a building, but *you* are the temple and the throne is your *heart,* you should make sure that the foundation of the heart is strictly the sacrificial, selfless devotion to God that is portrayed by Jesus throughout the Scripture. He was the Lamb led to slaughter, and He made it His life's work to let the world know that He loved the Father and did exactly what the Father wanted Him to do (John 14:31). With this as your foundation for everything in your life, you are as solid as the Rock you have founded your life upon. Nothing can bring you down!

Understand that your body is not your own. It has been designed as the dwelling place for the King. You are not the owner of your body—God is. You have no right to take one bite more than what He says. God is the CEO; you are, at best, the manager. For you to stay five to eighty pounds overweight year after year is not your right. God wants to rule among a group of people—the called out—a remnant willing to move their will aside and allow the holy personality of God to rule their lives. If God's will is on the throne of your heart, you will be holy (1 Peter 1:13–15). You will stumble, but as time goes by, you can experience more and more of His personality (Holy Spirit) ruling your life. This is the calling of the virgin bride of Christ (2 Cor. 11:2–4). In other words, we are being called back to Jesus' original teachings about the church in order to understand that it's a *spiritual* house once again, a *spiritual* house that can unify in defiance of brick and mortar.

We've gotten so far away from this teaching that the body of Christ is in a very ineffective and vulnerable state. It is a form of religion, but it is denying its power (1 Tim. 3:5). It is gathering in large buildings, but perhaps only a scattered few have the right foundation. There is as much lack of pure devotion to God *inside* most church buildings as outside the church buildings. Gallup polls tell us that approximately half the people in America attend these church buildings,[2] yet we have increasing divorce and crime rates and other problems. Thousands upon thousands continue to be killed by drunk drivers on our roads. Even though we are taking more antidepressants than ever recorded in the history of mankind, we are more unhappy than we've ever been. We buy more and do more things without the leading of God than ever before. Greed is at its zenith. Our lust for food is a defining characteristic of this country to the world. More children are overweight than ever before. Instances of the bizarre—such as self-mutilation, gang murders, and children committing suicide—are on the rise. We have lost up from down, truth from a lie, and we call darkness "light." The religious define *sin* as a thing rather than a motive of the heart of man. No wonder our children feel hopeless and so many contemplate ending their lives.

We could be mad at the government, but that's not who God is upset at. God is upset at a halfhearted grace message that has proved to be only a license to sin. Jude 4 says, "For certain men whose condemnation was written about long ago have secretly slipped in among you. They are godless men, who change the grace of our God into a license for immorality and deny Jesus Christ our only Sovereign and Lord." This Scripture was written for the leaders of today!

God's Word calls us to be holy. God's grace has enabled us to walk free of this sin. Our lack of repentance is confusing the church, and our continued shameful ways distort the way of truth of this gospel. The Apostle Peter wrote: "Many will follow their shameful ways and will bring the way of truth into disrepute" (2 Peter 2:2). Since we have so many buildings in this nation that have a form of religion but deny its power, it confuses the people inside the buildings and encourages those outside to think those inside are hypocrites. Who wants to believe the words preached by hypocrites? Why come to Christ if coming offers no way out for the prisoners? But the Bible says,

So I tell you this, and insist on it in the Lord, that you must no longer live as the Gentiles do, in the futility of their thinking. They are darkened in their understanding and separated from the life of God because of the ignorance that is in them due to the hardening of their hearts. Having lost all sensitivity, they have given themselves over to sensuality so as to indulge in every kind of impurity, with a continual lust for more. You, however, did not come to know Christ that way. Surely you heard of him and were taught in him in accordance with the truth that is in Jesus. You were taught, with regard to your former way of life, to put off your old self, which is being corrupted by its deceitful desires; to be made new in the attitude of your minds; and to put on the new self, created to be like God in true righteousness and holiness. Therefore each of you must put off falsehood and speak truthfully to his neighbor, for we are all members of one body. "In your anger do not sin": Do not let the sun go down while you are still angry, and do not give the devil a foothold. He who has been stealing must steal no longer, but must work, doing something useful with his own hands, that he may have something to share with those in need. Do not let any unwholesome talk come out of your mouths, but only what is helpful for building others up according to their needs, that it may benefit those who listen. And do not grieve the Holy Spirit of God, with whom you were sealed for the day of redemption. Get rid of all bitterness, rage and anger, brawling and slander, along with every form of malice. Be kind and compassionate to one another, forgiving each other, just as in Christ God forgave you. Be imitators of God, therefore, as dearly loved children and live a life of love, just as Christ loved us and gave himself up for us as a fragrant offering and sacrifice to God. But among you there must not be even a hint of sexual immorality, or of any kind of impurity, or of greed, because these are improper for God's holy people. *Nor should there be obscenity, foolish talk or coarse joking, which are out of place, but rather thanksgiving. For of this you can be sure: No immoral, impure or greedy person—such a man is an idolater—has any inheritance in the kingdom of Christ and of God. Let no one deceive you with empty words, for because of such things God's wrath comes on those who are disobedient.* (Eph. 4:17–5:6, emphasis added)

THE CHURCH IS EASILY MISLED

Being easily deceived and being misled were the defining characteristics of God's children from Eden to Jerusalem. The Apostle Paul wrote a letter to the saints in the city of Corinth,

I am jealous for you with a godly jealousy. I promised you to one husband, to Christ, so that I might present you as a pure virgin to him. But I am afraid that just as Eve was deceived by the serpent's cunning, your minds may somehow be led astray from your sincere and pure devotion to Christ. For if someone comes to you and preaches a Jesus other than the Jesus we preached, or if you receive a different spirit from the one you received, or a different gospel from the one you accepted, you put up with it easily enough. (2 Cor. 11:2–4, emphasis added)

We are no different from the called out in Corinth; we easily put up with false teachings. We are always looking for an easier new message.

And then in Galatians, Paul wrote: "The acts of the sinful nature are obvious. . . . I warn you, as I did before, that those who live like this will not inherit the kingdom of God" (Gal. 5:19a, 21b). Why did Paul say, "I warn you, as I did before"? After all, this message is clear and simple. You see, Satan's masterpiece lie is powerful and has only strengthened through the generations.

For of this you can be sure: No immoral, impure or greedy person—such a man is an idolater—has any inheritance in the kingdom of Christ and of God. Let no one deceive you with empty words. (Eph. 5:5–6a)

First John 1:5–6 says, "This is the message we have heard from him and declare to you: God is light; in him, there is no darkness at all. If we claim to have fellowship with him yet walk in the darkness, we lie and do not live by the truth." We lie to ourselves.

Remember what it says in 1 John 3:

> *Dear children, do not let anyone lead you astray. He who does what is right is righteous, just as he is righteous. He who does what is sinful is of the devil, because the devil has been sinning from the beginning. The reason the Son of God appeared was to destroy the devil's work. No one who is born of God will continue to sin, because God's seed remains in him; he cannot go on sinning, because he has been born of God. This is how we know who the children of God are and who the children of the devil are: Anyone who does not do what is right is not a child of God. (vv. 7–10a)*

We have strayed so far from the truth that we are more afraid to associate with someone who claims to let God rule his mind and heart (someone who is holy) than with someone who is living in adultery (someone who is of the devil). Laying down sin is not a *work*—it is essential and foundational for the kingdom of *God*. Jesus came to cast the devil out of our hearts and to replace him with God's Spirit.

And finally, the Bible says,

> To the Jews who had believed him, Jesus said, "If you hold to my teaching, you are really my disciples. Then you will know the truth, and the truth will set you free." They answered him, "We are Abraham's descendants and have never been slaves of anyone. How can you say that we shall be set free?" Jesus replied, "I tell you the truth, everyone who sins is a slave to sin. Now a slave has no permanent place in the family, but a son belongs to it forever. So if the Son sets you free, you will be free indeed." (John 8:31–36)

Jesus is saying that someone who continues in sin does not belong to the family of God, but sons are offspring who have the Father's eyes, attitude, walk, and heart, and sons belong to the kingdom forever.

Over the centuries, Satan has done major damage to the basic truth of the good news of Jesus Christ allowing people to call darkness "light" or say "you're okay continuing in sin." No—we just read that the Bible says, "Do not let anyone lead you astray. He who does what is right is righteous. . . . He who does what is sinful is of the devil" (1 John 3:7–8).

We cannot continue in sin. Yes, we all have sinned and we do stumble from time to time, but "continuing in sin" is an attitude of the heart that says to God, "I love the world more than You." That rebellious attitude will not enter the kingdom of God. If you continue in sin and know it, do you realize that it is the devil's work in you? Be fully warned! Over the centuries, because of this distorted teaching, we are more afraid to say "we are holy" than "we are sinners." We think that saying "we are sinners" is humble and "we are holy" is arrogant. But think again. . . . It is the opposite! To be afraid and to believe it is *not* your right to take what has not been given to you is humility.

Jesus told His disciples and listeners, "I tell you the truth, unless you eat the flesh of the Son of Man and drink his blood, you have no life in you" (John 6:53). The disciples knew that eating His flesh and drinking His blood was a metaphor implying that they should live the type of lifestyle that He lived and should do only the will of the Father every day. On hearing it, many of His disciples said, "This is a hard teaching. Who can accept it?" Aware that His disciples were perplexed by this, Jesus said to them, "Does this offend you?" And the Bible tells us that many of His disciples turned back then and did not follow Him (John 6:60–61, 66).

Yes, that teaching is hard, but the people reading this book happen to be the "called out." You have embraced these hard teachings and have found nothing but ecstatic joy from a Jesus who has taught you that life comes from death to self. Standing up for God's truth—that someone who is a slave to sin cannot enter the kingdom—may cause you to be hated in the world and to feel lonely. But everyone who has repented from overeating can testify to 1 John 5:3–4a, "This is love for God: to obey his commands. And his commands are not burdensome, for everyone born of God overcomes the world."

You may have come up against resistance to the teachings in Weigh Down† before. But if you have read this far, you understand the Holy Scripture when it says:

> It is God's will that you should be sanctified: that you should avoid sexual immorality; that each of you should learn to control his own body in a way that is holy and honorable, not in passionate lust like the heathen, who do not know God; and that in this matter no one should wrong his brother or take advantage of him. The Lord will punish men for all such sins, as we have already told you and warned you. For God did not call us to be impure, but to live a holy life. Therefore, he who rejects this instruction does not reject man but God, who gives you his Holy Spirit. (1 Thess. 4:3–8, emphasis added)

God did not call you to be impure, but to live a holy life. Abel knew that from the very beginning, but Cain always tried to get around this calling. The people who understand that Zion is God's *holy* hill and who want to live in Zion must be holy and humble—a contrite group (Isa. 66:2b). They must beat their breasts and call out to God for continual dependence on His Holy Spirit and the attitude of Christ. They must be continually putting their own will to death. Your will has less and less of a heartbeat as you journey along. Today, I feel freer than ever to wake up and ask, "God, what do You want me to do today?"

You have been given the ability to make this choice. Satan and his forces keep you confused. Satan tells you that it is okay to be the offspring of Cain, and that even though God does not like it, you will be accepted by God. To end the confusion, you must stay in the Word because God said the following: "If you do what is right, will you not be accepted? But if you do not do what is right, sin is crouching at your door; it desires to have you, but you must master it" (Gen. 4:7). The church run by the Cains of this world seems like the predominant church of the day, and it is the *counterfeit* church. Many gather every week to praise God and Jesus for ignoring the heart and seeing each person as sinless when each one is living in sin. I would jump up and down if that were true. But it is a lie.

I truly praise God for giving me the opportunity to repent—to turn—and leave room for His Holy Spirit to rule my life. My body is His temple. I praise Jesus Christ for forgiving this temple of all past sins and for times on this journey when my flesh takes over temporarily. How awesome to be forgiven of this!

The Old and New Testaments refer to Babylon as the antithesis of Israel. Israel, Zion, or the New Jerusalem refers to people free to love God with a sincere and pure heart. Pure means single-hearted. Matthew 5:48 quotes Jesus: "Be perfect, therefore, as your heavenly Father is perfect." So Jesus commands us to be perfect, and *perfect* means "whole." We are to be singly and wholly devoted to the true God. Now we can do this. People get upset with those terms because

I started Weigh Down† wanting to lose weight, but I gained so much more. God has restored the joy of my salvation, healed my marriage, and now our children have begun to model our eating behaviors. God has miraculously performed spiritual surgery on my heart, and He used Weigh Down† to change my entire life!
Tom & Donna Lucia-Downs—Centreville, MD
Tom lost 50 lbs.—Donna lost 86 lbs.

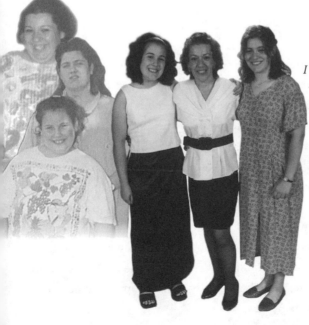

I can honestly say that Weigh Down† not only helped me lose weight, but it also saved my marriage and saved my soul. Thank You, Lord, for all of the love and happiness You have brought to my entire family.
The Celotto Family
Pequea, PA
Joanne, mother of 7
Lost 100+ lbs.
Annie, 13 years old
Lost 60+ lbs.
Marie, 20 years old
Lost 65 lbs.
All have kept
it off 2 years.

they have been distorted by Satan and made to be some unattainable terms that could apply to no one but God. God has simply asked us to have *one* God, just as He wants us to have one husband or wife. It works better if you have only one employer; otherwise, you will become devoted to one and despise the other. This is not a work— this is an ability that God gave Abel. God did not force Abel or Cain, yet Cain tried to get the approval without the single-minded, single-hearted devotion. That is the counterfeit church, and it is called Babylon. Every time God's children were steeped in rebellion and bent on following the Cains of the world, they would ignore the prophets who prophesied destruction and captivity. For example, the prophet Jeremiah was beaten and put in stocks, threatened with death, arrested and imprisoned in a dungeon, and thrown into a dry cistern to sink in the mud and starve, just to mention some of what he endured (Jer. 20:1–2; 26:8; 37:14b–16; 38:6b, 9b). The people from a synagogue where Jesus spoke even took Him to a hill overlooking the town and tried to push Him off a cliff (Luke 4:28–29).

You Are the Remnant

God means business, and we need to take an honest look at ourselves and the called out. Worship services could be a stench to His nostrils because the hearts are wrong. Counterfeit churches have a "safe grace" plan, or they are strict for man-made rules. The Apostle Paul said that he wouldn't allow these difficult, legalistic, non-heart-effective, distracting, man-made rules in for one moment (read Gal. 1–6). The true universal church, whether a home group, a small group, or a large number anywhere in any city, will teach strict heart lessons, and the foundation will be Jesus Christ. It will be made up of people who do not need to tell others they are Christian because they are so radically different, they are transformed—new creatures. The early Christians understood this message, and that is why fellowships were described as in these passages from Acts:

*Those who accepted his message were baptized, and about three thou-
sand were added to their number that day. They devoted themselves
to the apostles' teaching and to the fellowship, to the breaking of
bread and to prayer. Everyone was filled with awe, and many wonders and miraculous signs were done by the apostles. All the believers
were together and had everything in common. Selling their possessions and goods, they gave to anyone as he had need. Every day they
continued to meet together in the temple courts. They broke bread in
their homes and ate together with glad and sincere hearts, praising
God and enjoying the favor of all the people. And the Lord added to
their number daily those who were being saved.* (2:41–47)

*After they prayed, the place where they were meeting was shaken.
And they were all filled with the Holy Spirit and spoke the word of
God boldly. All the believers were one in heart and mind. No one
claimed that any of his possessions was his own, but they shared
everything they had. With great power the apostles continued to testify to the resurrection of the Lord Jesus, and much grace was upon
them all. There were no needy persons among them. For from time to
time those who owned lands or houses sold them, brought the money
from the sales and put it at the apostles' feet, and it was distributed
to anyone as he had need.* (4:31–35)

Three thousand people came to the Lord in one day. They didn't
praise God and Jesus for letting them live in sin—they praised God
for getting them out of their prisons of serving the fleshly desires.

All along, God has looked for a faith in His abilities and His decisions and His coordination—a faith that would understand putting
a knife up to your own child as Abraham did. A faith that would
build an ark in the middle of nowhere. A faith like Noah's that would
not side against God for destroying the wicked. All along, God has
looked for a group of people who had such a faith that it would come
through into their actions because the Bible tells us,

You foolish man, do you want evidence that faith without deeds is use-less? Was not our ancestor Abraham considered righteous for what he did when he offered his son Isaac on the altar? You see that his faith and his actions were working together, and his faith was made complete by what he did. And the scripture was fulfilled that says, "Abraham believed God, and it was credited to him as righteousness," and he was called God's friend. You see that a person is justified by what he does and not by faith alone. (James 2:20–24, emphasis added)

"THE CALLED OUT"

Flee from Babylon! Run for your lives! Do not be destroyed because of her sins. It is time for the LORD's vengeance; he will pay her what she deserves. Babylon was a gold cup in the LORD's hand; she made the whole earth drunk. The nations drank her wine; therefore they have now gone mad. (Jer. 51:6–7)

Much of the church has become drunk with the "safe grace" message. People are numb to warnings and can't see the danger of driving ninety miles per hour down the wrong side of the street. We need to sober up.

"Come, I will show you the punishment of the great prostitute, who sits on many waters. With her the kings of the earth committed adultery and the inhabitants of the earth were intoxicated with the wine of her adulteries." . . . *This title was written on her forehead:*

> *MYSTERY BABYLON THE GREAT*
> *THE MOTHER OF PROSTITUTES*
> *AND OF THE ABOMINATIONS OF THE EARTH. . . .*

After this I saw another angel coming down from heaven. He had great authority, and the earth was illuminated by his splendor. With a mighty voice he shouted: "Fallen! Fallen is Babylon the Great! She has become a home for demons and a haunt for every evil spirit, a haunt for every unclean and detestable bird. For all the nations have drunk the maddening wine of her adulteries. The kings of the earth committed adultery with her, and the merchants of the earth grew rich from her excessive luxuries." Then I heard another voice from heaven say: "Come out of her, my people, so that you will not share in her sins, so that you will not receive any of her plagues; for her sins are piled up to heaven." (Rev. 17:1b–2, 5; 18:1–5a)

When God calls you out of Babylon—that is, the counterfeit church or religion, or the world—to be different and to be holy (a holy priesthood), it may not always be easy to obey. It may not be a teaching that is readily accepted by people who don't feel that holiness is required in our actions. Remember, Noah had to face the cruel remarks of skeptical, wicked people who would tell him that he didn't need to build an ark. Those same people would later witness the ark being lifted high above the earth, and the righteous would witness the wicked being drowned. God has called you to this same faith. You are the called out, or a remnant of righteousness. You must unify with the "called out" and build an ark—a stand against sin.

Contemplate the unique, called-out life of Noah, who stayed focused on the will of God and separated himself from Babylon (or the wicked). Noah and his family floated on the waters for 150 days. Then God sent a great wind over the earth, and the waters receded steadily from the earth. The Bible tells us, "At the end of the hundred and fifty days the water had gone down, and on the seventeenth day of the seventh month the ark came to rest on the mountains of Ararat" (Gen. 8:3b–4). The tops of the mountains eventually became visible.

After forty days Noah opened the window he had made in the ark and sent out a raven, and it kept flying back and forth until the water had dried up from the earth. Then he sent out a dove to see if the water had receded from the surface of the ground. But the dove could find no place to set its feet because there was water over all the surface of the earth; so it returned to Noah in the ark. He reached out his hand and took the dove and brought it back to himself in the ark. He waited seven more days and again sent out the dove from the ark. When the dove returned to him in the evening, there in its beak was a freshly plucked olive leaf! Then Noah knew that the water had receded from the earth. . . . Noah then removed the covering from the ark and saw that the surface of the ground was dry. . . . Then God said to Noah, "Come out of the ark, you and your wife and your sons and their wives. Bring out every kind of living creature that is with you . . . so they can multiply on the earth and be fruitful." (Gen. 8:6–11, 13b, 15–17)

The remnant was starting over.

Noah built an altar to the Lord, taking some of all the clean animals and clean birds, and he sacrificed the burnt offering. The Lord smelled the pleasing aroma and said, "Never again will all life be cut off by the waters of a flood; never again will there be a flood to destroy the earth" (Gen. 9:11b). And God gave the rainbow as a sign of this covenant. And this remnant, who had trusted in the God of the Flood, found it very easy to trust in the God of the rainbow.

Noah could have been overwhelmed by this experience. He could have given up on many occasions. He could have quit fifty years into building an ark that seemed to be an endless project. He could have been disheartened at the continual barrage of comments about the futility of serving God. He could have been overwhelmed by the job of feeding two of every creature. He could have lost his composure on the third day of the Flood when a massive number of bodies were floating on the water, drowned—on the twentieth day of rain, when it seemed as if God's anger would not relent—and on the one-hundredth day of floating on the water with no sign of land.

But no—he loved God so much that his first response was to offer a sacrifice of clean animals to God. Noah could have begged God not to be so hard on the wicked, or he could have questioned God and asked Him, "Why sacrifice the clean animals? Why couldn't I sacrifice the unclean?" But Hebrews 11:7 says, "By faith Noah, when warned about things not yet seen, in *holy fear* built an ark to save his family. By his faith he condemned the world and became heir of the righteousness that comes by faith" (italics added).

One man's faith can condemn many people today. Noah is only one man of great faith in Hebrews 11, and he stands among Abel, Abraham, Moses, and Rahab. He stands among Samson, David, Samuel, and the prophets. About the people of faith, the writer of Hebrews said,

> *Others were tortured and refused to be released, so that they might gain a better resurrection. Some faced jeers and flogging, while still others were chained and put in prison. They were stoned; they were sawed in two; they were put to death by the sword. . . . Therefore, since we are surrounded by such a great cloud of witnesses, let us throw off everything that hinders and the sin that so easily entangles, and let us run with perseverance the race marked out for us.* (Heb. 11:35b–37a; 12:1)

We are surrounded by a great cloud of witnesses who are cheering us on, letting us know that God has provided everything we need for life, godliness, holiness, and a pure life without greed, adultery, or idolatry (2 Peter 1:3). I also know that I am among a faithful group who are, by their very lives, walking in the light and putting off the old and putting on the new (Eph. 4:22–24). A group of people who would never call darkness "light" and confuse the people. A group of people who would never distort the Word of God and Jesus Christ (2 Cor. 4:2). I am honored to be among the faithful and the called out reading these words. If you have taken to heart this message of repentance, then you have separated yourself from man. Let us commit to God today to throw off everything that hinders and the sin that so easily entangles. Let us all help each other run with perseverance this race that's clearly marked out for us—the New Jerusalem, the Remnant—as Jesus is at the threshing floor, separating the wheat from the chaff, the good from the evil.

WE ARE NOT OUR OWN

In conclusion, may we all learn from history that God is a God of love. But may we live (and approach our food or any other idol) as if we know—really know—there will be a Judgment Day, a kicking from Paradise, a burning of sin at Sodom and Gomorrah, a flood on the wicked, a death for the disobedient in the desert, a destruction of the rebellion in Jerusalem, and a Final Judgment of all mankind. God means business. Seriously consider the state of your heart and enter the ark of the righteous remnant—the called out—and float above the world with the righteous.

Read the description of the church as found in 1 Corinthians 3:10–17. As noted earlier, your body is not your own. You are not the creator of your body. You are not the boss of your body. Supposedly, God is on the throne of your heart, and your body is the dwelling place of the King. What makes you think you have the right to destroy it by overeating? What makes you think you have the right to eat beyond what your body is calling for? It's not your body to destroy. This Scripture points out that God will destroy anyone who destroys His temple. Contemplate this foundational perspective until you can say with Job, "Naked I came from my mother's womb, and naked I will depart" (Job 1:21a), knowing that we don't deserve anything and whatever we have is from God. If you will concentrate on this thought for the rest of your life, you, like Jesus, will "not consider equality with God something to be grasped" (Phil. 2:6b), and you will not continue in overindulging, for God loves you so much.

What You Can Do Today

- Go where God is leading you in Scripture.

- *Endeavor to be holy.* God's Word calls us to be holy. Do not deny the power of the Lord; He offers *complete* freedom for those enslaved to the world. Keep a list of Scriptures that reference our call to holiness.

- *Identify false teachers.* God's true messengers call His chosen people to embrace the hard teachings of Jesus and to find joy, peace, and love in dying to self. False teachers offer an easier message, saying, "It's okay to continue in sin." The path to the Father is not always smooth. Stay in the Word so you will be battle ready.

- *Rid your life of idols.* Wipe away the idols that separate you from God and His grace. Clean up the litter filling your heart, so you can experience God's complete fulfillment and love.

- *Prepare for judgment.* Noah and the people of his age were warned of the impending disaster. Look for signs around you that God is warning His "called out" to get ready for judgment.

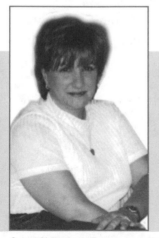

I have given up many things in my 34 years, such as drugs, cigarettes, pornography, and alcohol, but I have struggled fiercely with food. I started Weigh Down† in 1994 and lost weight, only to put it all back on. Several halfhearted measures failed and left me discouraged again. Then I saw the EXODUS from Strongholds promotional video and cried. It was as if the Lord was saying, "You can have victory again!" I began the classes, and the weight has started coming off again. The Lord's grace is so good—to forgive me and allow me success after I flirted with the devil again.
Susan Sizemore-LaPorte—Pewaukee, WI

Susan Sizemore-LaPorte asserts that halfhearted surrender will not lead to success.

Be My Guest

I love to be a servant to guests at dinner parties in my home. In the summer, it is not uncommon to find my husband grilling steaks, hamburgers, and spicy hot dogs. The food is not the focus. Instead, there is plenty of love and fellowship. As you transfer your focus off the food and onto God, you will find that many of your old habits are no longer there because you have risen above focusing on and loving the food. Your heart, your mind, and your soul are focused entirely on loving the Father. In the past when you invited guests over for dinner, you may have saved the best meat cuts for yourself. How? Perhaps by hiding the biggest and juiciest steak or hamburger at the bottom of the pile. You even had the tendency to "strong-arm" your way to the front of the buffet line, or you may have hidden some foods until you were ready to serve yourself. But now, you are no longer interested in serving yourself first—you live to serve God and others. You want your guests to have the very best portions because the food no longer has a grip on you. In fact, you receive a blessing each time you serve the best portions to your guests. This blessing might be a compliment about how good the food tastes or how much your guests have enjoyed the gathering. Your focus has shifted from the food onto loving the Father and doing exactly what He wants. You have learned how to get your will out of the way so that you can do His will and serve others with a cheerful heart. At most parties, I am so tired from serving that I am too tired to eat! I fix a plate, cover it up, and set it aside to eat after all the guests have left that night or even the next day. Serving God and His people was my food.

fourteen

HEAVEN'S KISS

Many people do well the first few weeks, but when they realize that God really expects them to eat less food, the heat of the testing can melt their spirit. They want out of this hot test of self-denial.

Over the years, one of the basic truths I've tried to teach people was to look at life from God's perspective. In fact, my major motivation for going into work every day is not only to combat the inaccurate opinions that people have of God, but also to make people aware of what a rotten deal God has received. For instance, it's almost embarrassing that we need a good motivational sermon to lay our idols down. I can't really fathom why we're not selling everything we have for this relationship with God. Many people don't see how good we have it and how great He is. We don't see how arrogant we are by expecting so much from Him. It's almost as if God is on trial, and if He's "good enough," we'll think about giving Him *some* of the time in our day and *some* of our hearts, a *portion* of our passion, and a *bit* of our souls. I feel a pain deep inside every time I see His side of the story or contemplate how He must feel, knowing that He is the Creator and Sustainer of all.

A CREATOR HAS HIS RIGHTS

It is now my heart's desire to think about God all the time and to offer Him all that I have. I trust in *all* His decisions, and there is

absolutely *nothing* about God that I want to change. I believe that He
needs to hear us say that. I am sure that His feelings are hurt that
more people don't just automatically adore Him and trust Him. I
love the God who sends blessings, but I love the disciplining God as
well. I understand and respect the God who sent the great Flood and
the devastating plagues. A Creator has His rights, and I don't have
any problem with a Creator who can—with a single word—create
life or destroy life. I love God, for I see all that He does and define
Him as a God of love. I don't want Him to change. I don't want Him
to think that we want Him to offer more food, more money, more
justice, more grace, or more love than He
already has. I don't want God to think that
I want Him to change His personality or
His justice system or His laws. So many
people want to remake God. They love the
heaven and the blessing part of His personality, but they do not respect and
understand the essential decision of hell
for the hearts that show contempt for
their Maker. I love Him for *everything,* and
I do not bleed over any tough decisions He makes—from stirring up
wars and plagues, to sending His own Son to a torturous death. I
pray that He never, ever changes.

A Creator has His rights, and I don't have any problem with a Creator who can—with a single word—create life or destroy life.

Jesus warned us that in the end times, "because of the increase of
wickedness, the love of most will grow cold, but he who stands firm
to the end will be saved" (Matt. 24:12–13). I believe that God has been
warning me to warn all people that because of the lack of acceptance
of Him and His rules to live by, we are under judgment from God
right now. We need to examine the light that is within and make sure
that there is no darkness. Just as the Israelites put the blood of the
lamb over every door, we must be sure that it is Jesus' blood that we
depend upon—blood that denies self, blood that is constantly using
its mind and strength to ask God what He wants today, blood that is

carrying out His instructions. That is the bloodline that ran through our Savior, and the blood that He asked us to drink (John 6). But Jesus warned us all that in the end times, the love of most would grow cold. It is very important to keep the flame for God alive.

Some of us need a blood transfusion. In fact, that was the very problem that the church in the city of Ephesus had. Revelation 2 says,

> *I know your deeds, your hard work and your perseverance. I know that you cannot tolerate wicked men, that you have tested those who claim to be apostles but are not, and have found them false. You have persevered and have endured hardships for my name, and have not grown weary. Yet I hold this against you: You have forsaken your first love. Remember the height from which you have fallen! Repent and do the things you did at first. If you do not repent, I will come to you and remove your lampstand from its place. . . . He who has an ear, let him hear what the Spirit says to the churches.* (vv. 2–5, 7a)

We have talked much in this book about looking out for the false pastors of the day—and like the church in Ephesus, you may have done this—but have you lost your first, honeymoon-passionate love? Yes, you can identify and refuse to tolerate all of the false teachers, and that will help

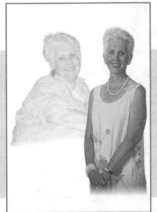

I've lost about 50 pounds with Weigh Down†. God has truly done an awesome job in reshaping me. What an awesome Creator we have! God has shown me how much He loves me, teaching me to trust Him and fall in love with Him more each day. I've also realized that when I am truly in love with Him, my love spills over, and I am anxious and excited about what He asks me to do. I give Him all the praise, glory, and credit.
Debi Gick—Lake Forest, CA

Debi Gick discovered the amazing love that God has for her when she turned to Him instead of the food.

the body of Christ—God is going to praise you for this. However, if you lose the passion for your first love, you have lost everything.

THE JACKET STORY

There was a time several months before I wrote this book that was very frightening for me because I felt as if I was losing my foothold of my relationship with God. I call this the "Jacket Story." Love grows, or love dies. The fact is that I had been unaware that I was not as passionate for God and Jesus as I had been. The "Jacket Story" is a story of embracing the entire cross that we have been given in life, and no one has described this embrace more than Jesus Christ through His thirty-three-year walk on earth.

Love is such a mystery. The Apostle Paul put this heart condition into action verbs in the letter to the church—those who were called out to follow Christ—in Corinth. You know this letter as 1 Corinthians and the passage as chapter 13. Paul was inspired to say that love is the greatest of all gifts, and that we should all pursue it and desire it. But anyone, and especially God, can see through you if it is not real, just as old wine and new wine do not mix. Jealousy, malice, hate, slander, bad feelings, apathy, antiauthority, and the inability to submit are all the antithesis of love. Now, if you have bad feelings toward and absolutely hate *injustice*, that's not what I'm talking about. Defending God's position is righteousness and love. Don't be confused. But true love will not come across as a resounding gong or a clanging cymbal. It will be sincerely selfless and fearlessly outgoing. It will be genuine.

To the called out in Corinth, Paul poured out his heart, teaching:

> *If I speak in the tongues of men and of angels, but have not love, I am only a resounding gong or a clanging cymbal. If I have the gift of prophecy and can fathom all mysteries and all knowledge, and if I have a faith that can move mountains, but have not love, I am noth-*

ing. If I give all I possess to the poor and surrender my body to the flames, but have not love, I gain nothing. Love is patient, love is kind. It does not envy, it does not boast, it is not proud. It is not rude, it is not self-seeking, it is not easily angered, it keeps no record of wrongs. Love does not delight in evil but rejoices with the truth. It always protects, always trusts, always hopes, always perseveres. Love never fails. . . . And now these three remain: faith, hope, and love. But the greatest of these is love. (1 Cor. 13:1–8a, 13)

So faith in God and hope in God are great—but the greatest of these is love for God. We must always remember that this love must be for God first, and then it will automatically flow to mankind second. But when your love grows cold, if you are gifted but lack love, if you have forsaken your first love, then you are nothing and you have nothing.

What started off in October with the purchase of a jacket might seem to you a minor thing, but it represented much, much more. First of all, you have to understand that I was taking a vacation just because I looked at the world and saw everybody else taking vacations. I started wondering if my children were needing more exposure or more retreats. Surely, God wanted us to work more of these into our lives. But because I did more assuming and less inquiring of God, He did not bless the weekend trip to Boston at all. The first day there, I went shopping. I thought I would try to catch up on what the world got to do all the time—shop. What happened was that I had purchased several items for my family upstairs in the department store, and then I found two items for me downstairs. One item I didn't need at all—a very expensive suit jacket—but I could use it for a talk that I was going to do in front of one thousand very well-dressed women in my hometown. The other item I felt that I needed—a ski jacket. You have to realize that when I believed the world was passing me by, not only did I jump in there and plan a trip to Boston, I planned our first ski trip to Utah in January. We were going for four days to see what the world was raving about.

This attitude of feeling sorry for my life because I never took a vacation seemed justified. Not only was I wrong about that, but I didn't realize something even more grave—God was gearing up for action in His kingdom while I was looking for retirement. I was missing God's leading. As the psalmist said,

> Surely God is good to Israel,
>   to those who are pure in heart.
> But as for me, my feet had almost slipped;
>   I had nearly lost my foothold.
> For I envied the arrogant
>   when I saw the prosperity [vacations] of the wicked. (Ps. 73:1–3)

The credit card went through when I purchased the items for my family upstairs. But when I went downstairs to purchase my jackets, the credit card would not go through. Not thinking that it was a warning from God, I used another credit card. That evening, while we were eating dinner and discussing the credit cards, I told my family that I was very put out with the bank. I finally had a chance to shop, and now I didn't have access to any money. Michael said, "Well, what makes you think that God just didn't want you to have the jacket?" Well, that's just great. That's exactly what you get when you bring up your kids in the Lord.

My Foot Was Slipping

As soon as it came out of his mouth, it hit my heart like a ton of bricks. Michael was exactly right. Later that evening, I was not only awakened in the night with some heavy-duty Scriptures from God, but He also struck me with an illness that caused me to lose my voice. It was gone for almost a month, and I had not been sick for nearly three years. On top of that, one fingernail after another started to break to the quick. This was significant and very frightening to me.

Before Weigh Down[†], I was known as "Fatman" or "Fatboy." My mom is a nurse and she made me eat fat-free and low-fat foods, and they didn't work. But after Weigh Down[†], I feel 10 million times better and I feel like a real kid!

**Matthew Raulston
Claremore, OK
12 years old
Lost 22 lbs.**

I started going to Weigh Down[†] with my mom because I was tired of the way I looked and I just decided to make a change. I felt like I was doing something good for myself. I learned that my body is a temple of the Holy Spirit and I can't do what I want to do with it, but I have to do what God wants me to do.

**Alexandra Isaac—St. Louis, MO
14 years old
Lost 40 lbs.**

When I joined Weigh Down[†], I didn't believe I would be able to do it. But through God's grace, I not only dropped 7 dress sizes, but I also lost a very bad attitude. I never imagined I would be where I am today. I can't wait to see what the Lord has in store for me.

**Heather Ritter
Bedford, IN
18 years old
Lost 78 lbs.**

I didn't think I was ever going to lose weight. I always compared myself to others and I found myself having a hatred toward them. But God showed me that I would lose the weight if I would reach toward Him and be what He wants me to be. Through Weigh Down[†], God has taught me to be obedient to Him and He has changed me.

**Jessica Boatwright—Marion, IN
16 years old
Lost 60 lbs.**

Before you think that breaking fingernails is a judgment sign from God for you, you have to understand that that was just something between me and God. You would have to understand that I had prayed to God more than a year before and asked Him for even stronger nails so that I could help convince His people of His good health plan. I don't really care that much about my nails. I rarely get manicures, and I rarely paint them anymore—I just don't take the time. But because I felt that healthy nails would glorify God, I prayed for them. Lo and behold, God made my nails healthier, stronger, and longer than they had ever been without splitting or breaking. My point is not to teach you to pray for long nails, but I can testify that your prayers will be answered if they have the right motive!

Every aspect of your life should glorify God and His truths so that people will know Him. There are many things that are secret agreements between me and God besides the fingernails, and one of them that applies to this story is my boxwoods. Two years ago, I had transplanted some eighty-year-old boxwoods. I just prayed over those boxwoods because I was advised by experts that it is nearly impossible to transplant large, old plants. God answered my prayers and did the extraordinary by blessing those boxwoods! They lived, and they put out new growth. These ten- to fifteen-foot boxwoods were successfully transplanted.

Well, now not only was I sick and had broken nails, but when I got home from Boston, I noticed that all of my boxwoods looked as if they might be dying. Their leaves were turning orange. My heart was broken, not because I cared about my nails or the boxwoods, but because they were secret prayer requests that kept me in touch with my relationship with God. As I ran my fingers over every missing nail, I knew I did not care about my nails—I wanted to be in good with God. I was dying inside, and I could not even concentrate on any conversations. I only went through the motions for the rest of the vacation. I scrambled every minute I could to find time with God, whose anger and judgment I felt. All I wanted to do was to get away from people and find God's approval again, no matter what it took. No longer was I interested in anything the world could offer. I had gone on vacation to see what I was missing and realized that I had had everything; but it was slipping away.

Galatians 6 says, "Do not be deceived: God cannot be mocked. A man reaps what he sows. The one who sows to please his sinful nature, from that nature will reap destruction; the one who sows to please the Spirit, from the Spirit will reap eternal life" (vv. 7–8). My foot had slipped—but my loving God was warning me. From the moment I realized that He was upset with me, I was committed to doing everything that I needed to do—and more—to get my relationship with my Alpha and Omega back up to speed. I started digging for silver.

As the Scripture says,

> And if you call out for insight
> and cry aloud for understanding,
> and if you look for it as for silver
> and search for it as for hidden treasure,
> then you will understand the fear of the LORD
> and find the knowledge of God. (Prov. 2:3–5)

I prayed and cried the rest of that night in Boston. I was desperate for a sign that God would not give me what I deserved, but would let me repent and get my foothold back—and replace what I had lost. I have friends, children, a husband, and all kinds of relationships; I know how hard it is to get back the exact relationship you had after you have lost trust in someone. I never expected that I could ever get the position back that I had. I just wanted to make sure that He wasn't totally rejecting me. Remember, when I first started off

I was committed to doing everything that I needed to do—and more—to get my relationship with my Alpha and Omega back up to speed.

with this relationship, I asked only that I could just be somewhere in heaven with God. As long as it was God's domain, I would settle for the humblest spot, way back in the back pasture. As the years have gone by, I would want to inch closer into God's actual castle. I would be willing to clean commodes—just let me be closer to His presence. But now, I was hoping that He would just not reject me totally. I knew that this wasn't just about overshopping. This was more about being complacent, envying the wicked, and missing the fact that God had a lot more work to be done in His kingdom. To you, it may seem to be a very small thing that the credit card didn't go through and I broke a few nails. But praise God, I have grown a little more sensitive over the years, and remember—these were private issues between me and God. I pray that I never miss the little and big signs God uses to warn me that I am going the wrong way.

GOD IS MERCIFUL

The first sign I asked for to show that God would accept me back was for Him to allow me to return the jacket that I knew I didn't need. I prayed that they had not already altered it. I now hated this jacket that was standing between me and God. You have to understand that this was a very prestigious store, and I don't like to return an item even to a mom-and-pop gasoline station. It's embarrassing! If you decided to take it out of the store, you really ought not to be so cavalier—you ought to keep it. I went into the store and faced the salesclerks. Unfortunately, they were all free and just staring at me like vultures. I prayed hard. The salesclerk took my ticket and went to the alterations department. After some time, she returned and said, "Mrs. Shamblin . . . [and my heart stopped beating], there has been some kind of mistake. We have not been able to alter your jacket and it's not ready. We have your address

I pray that I never miss the little and big signs God uses to warn me that I am going the wrong way.

so we will just mail it to you." Yes! God is so merciful. This gave me hope that I was going to be able to get out from underneath some of the consequences of my sin. Now for the hard part. I had to tell this commission-paid salesclerk that I was returning this expensive jacket, and at the same time try not to act so excited about it. I said something like this: "Well, I've been praying all weekend about this jacket, and I do not feel at peace about it. In other words, I do not feel that God wants me to buy this jacket." The well-dressed Bostonian salesclerk said, "Excuse me?" She did not understand this. Finally, she accepted the return. I was floating out of the store with only the ski jacket in my hands. At the time, it never occurred to me that God wanted me to return the ski jacket, too. How could I miss that?

Let's talk about this other vacation (not endorsed by God) to Utah—"the place to ski." They have snow in *October* at eight and nine thousand feet in Utah—much more in *January!* But as it turned out, God was not through with me. Little did the ski resorts know that when they let me come to Utah, I was bringing a curse with me. I was like Jonah on a ship to a place where he was not supposed to go. It would have been better for them if they had thrown me overboard! The curse was that it was the warmest week in January in the history of Utah. I have had to deal with this kind of thing before. One time, I was scheduled for Minnesota, and it was the coldest day in the history of that state. The temperature reading was fifty-seven to sixty degrees below zero. The windchill was worse! The jet well was frozen shut, so our jet not only had to land on ice, but also taxi to a jet well that would open. Your nose hairs froze immediately upon walking outside. But for this very cold Minnesota Date in the Desert, four hundred hearts still showed up to feed on God's Word and the power of His truth through testimonies. But as Minnesota was a test from God, Utah was a judgment from God.

Utah was fifty-seven to sixty degrees, even at eight thousand feet. Again, the warmest day in January in the history of Utah. The snow was literally melting out from underneath the ski slopes. It was a very

difficult surface to learn on because it was so slippery. But what's
more, when I got to Utah, I realized that I had left my new ski jacket
in Nashville! That was strange because I just knew I had packed it.
Even if I'd left it in Nashville—I could have it shipped overnight. The
Weigh Down† staff searched the entire house but said the jacket was
nowhere to be found. I reluctantly concluded the jacket had been
stolen out of my bags by the airline's employees. What are the odds
of that? I went to twenty-three cities on the book tour, and nothing
had ever been stolen out of my bags. Out of all the bags, why that bag
and why that jacket? It was definitely God, and I was crushed all over
again and getting very insecure. *Why can't I get this straight? What am
I doing wrong? Does He not want me to shop at all?* Thank goodness that
you do not really need a jacket when it is fifty-seven degrees outside.
(By the way, by the grace of God I learned to ski, and I managed to
inch my way down the slopes. I did get off the ski lifts—with help—
but God did not let me have the thrill everyone else in the world must
be having from skiing. It was just not going to be for me.)

Once again, this had little to do with overshopping or vacations.
This was much more involved than that. In the beginning of this dis-
ciplinary action by God, all I saw was my sin. I spent all my heart,
all my soul, all my mind, and all my strength reexamining everything
God could possibly want from me and making every effort to please
Him. As time went by, I eventually got my voice back, and my nails
slowly became strong again. I finally found a botanist who confirmed that the boxwoods were indeed living and could be nourished
back to good shape with fertilizer, pruning, and plenty of water.

This had nothing to do with God being strict with clothing. This
was God shaking me out of complacency. This was a strong wake-up
call that I was taking our relationship for granted—that I felt I had
done the job for Weigh Down†, but now it was time to retire. God was
in the process of calling the world into judgment, and I was out shopping or trying to vacation when He was busy with kingdom work. I
began to see the bigger picture. God was wanting to take this strong,

serious judgment and repentance message far beyond our relationship and to the body of Christ as a whole. Since judgment is under way, the church members and leaders need to repent *now*—not tomorrow.

Micah 3:1 says, "Listen, you leaders of Jacob, you rulers of the house of Israel. Should you not know justice?" God is saying that the leaders should know good from evil. We should know that it is not the food, the alcohol, or the drug that is evil—it is the *heart* of man! God has given us time to learn His ways, and He has presented this message of truth about good and evil, repentance, and the cross of Christ. But many a person distorts and hangs on to a complacent relationship that does not go all the way. We need to take this relationship with God and His kingdom more seriously and join the war on God's side—for good against evil. We should all purify ourselves with His Word and the blood of Christ. We should be battle ready for the days to come. God is warning us that this is no time to retire or to become complacent with this love relationship with Him. We should go into all the world and bring mankind the whole truth of the good news. We should let people know that Jesus is at the threshing floor and that He is taking His winnowing fork in His hands to gather the wheat into His barn and to burn the chaff with unquenchable fire. Since in the end, the love of most will grow cold, do all that you can to secure your heart to heaven!

I do know for a fact that before the Boston trip, I had been an extremely appreciative person for everything that God has done. I was like Job, a good man who knew he had done good things and knew of his relationship with God, but once God shook him up, Job said, "My ears had heard of you but now my eyes have seen you. Therefore I despise myself and repent in dust and ashes" (Job 42:5–6). My eyes had been opened, and I realized that there was a tremendous need for my complete attentiveness and purity before the Father, as well as being highly attuned to kingdom work—and God is very busy right now.

I realized that just like the boxwoods coming back to life with pruning, fertilizer, extra water, and effort, I could get this relationship back with God. I could then use what I had learned to warn, admonish, and exhort the body of Christ. The fruit of what I have learned has already challenged me and many others to get more into the Word. We are more serious with our opportunity to run like an athlete for the prize. I would trade nothing in the world for the disciplining hand of God because of the harvest of righteousness and a closer relationship. I had no idea that laying down the last ten pounds of worldly devotion would provide this much happiness and peace and purpose. I am happier now than I have ever, ever been because I feel so redirected and purposefully motivated to lay my life down for the bride of Christ.

I recommend wholeheartedly laying down everything you can possibly think of that is not exactly what the Father wants you to do. I'm a very happy slave to righteousness. Losing nails and boxwoods was enough to scare the life out of me. I would never choose to do anything now that would jeopardize abiding in Jesus Christ. Jesus said,

I am the vine; you are the branches. If a man remains in me and I in him, he will bear much fruit; apart from me you can do nothing. If anyone does not remain in me, he is like a branch that is thrown away and withers; such branches are picked up, thrown into the fire and burned. If you remain in me and my words remain in you, ask whatever you wish, and it will be given you. This is to my Father's glory, that you bear much fruit, showing yourselves to be my disciples. (John 15:5–8)

In Luke 10, Jesus said, "Martha, Martha, . . . you are worried and upset about many things, but only one thing is needed. Mary has chosen what is better, and it will not be taken away from her" (vv. 41–42). Jesus summed it up. Many things in this world get your attention and there are many good things to do, but only one is needed—living and fighting for this relationship, which includes fighting for the kingdom of Jesus Christ and God with all you are.

THE SONG

When I repented and got things straight with the Father, I felt that He was accepting me back. I got down on my knees and asked the Father for a song—a signature song—of my relationship with Him. Within fifteen minutes, He had given me the words and the tune to "Heaven's Kiss." The words of this song are based upon an event that happened several years ago. It was a time in my life that we were moving, and we were looking for a new place to live. I had been intensely in prayer every day for what the Lord wanted because I knew the God of the universe assigns a place and a time for each man. As it says in Acts 17:26, "From one man he made every nation of men, that they should inhabit the whole earth; and he determined the times set for them and the exact places where they should live." We know that God is involved in every detail of our relationship with Him and every detail of our lives.

I was very intense as I fell asleep that night. I couldn't believe that He was being so good to us with this move. During the wee hours of the morning, I dreamed that I looked up into heaven and blew God a kiss. As I was still looking up into heaven, I felt the wind blow and sweep around me. I felt that God was blowing me a kiss back, and all I can describe to you is that it was way beyond what I would expect to feel. It was a head-to-toe tingling sensation and electrifying sensation that did not stop—unlike anything I have ever felt. It was so powerful that I woke up—crying—for I had experienced something that at the time I felt that I should never, ever share with anyone, for it was between me and God. I had felt heaven's kiss.

Well, Boston was a spanking from heaven. So I have felt heaven's spanking *and* heaven's kiss—*both* acts of love from the Lord. I think it is interesting—just another one of God's ironies—that the song God gave me after *disciplining* me was "Heaven's Kiss." It was one thing to find out that I loved God when He was providing me a house, but it was a deeper experience that I found out that I loved

Him when He punished me. I learned deep in my heart that I would die for God—a wild experience to feel that feeling. I remember saying that there was nothing I wouldn't do to get His love.

I have learned that the only thing to fear is when God turns His face from you. There are about a dozen Scripture passages about God being so angry that He turns His face away. I felt a few moments of this. I feel certain that judgment is under way, and I indeed began to get this feeling in Boston. I was tested over a four-month period. I examined every possible attitude, unpleasant thought, or thoughtless word, and I chose to repent and get rid of every piece of dirt. When the storm blew to see what was in my heart, I felt that my house had been built upon the rock of Jesus Christ. The Rock of all that matters is wanting to do God's will. I discovered a heart grounded on accepting the sweet blessing from God as well as the hard walk of suffering ahead for those who obey Him. This is big!

Do you remember the story in Matthew 7:24–27 about the house built on the rock and the house built on sand? Sand has no depth or strength. When you build on the rock of Jesus Christ (meaning suffering, death to self, selflessness, humility, expecting nothing from God), then you are joyful and happy in God. Your foundation is a rock that is worth building on and that will not fall. Sand has faulty expectations and demands, and counts on a grace that allows the heart to continue in sin. The sand says, "God wants you happy," meaning "God wants your flesh happy." This is a lie and a false foundation. You are leaning on a broken reed.

As I was going through this purifying process of repentance and confession, Jesus washed me clean, just as He promises in 1 John 1:7. I do not want to ever be lax again, for I have tasted heaven's affection and heaven's rejection. They are far apart, and I will sell everything to run the race set before me and to talk others into a holy life that never looks to the left or the right. I pray that you are grounded on the rock of Jesus, a Rock that loves the Father who hands you a cross to carry. If you found you have a heart that has experienced its own "Jacket Story," and you realized that you, too, hate the world—in fact, you can't wait to return the world and exchange it for this relationship of love and cross-filled servanthood, and all you want is God's approval—then you are the house built on the rock and not on the sand. The houses that are built on the sand are going to fall because God's judgment is a powerful storm that is blowing right now on all those who have built on man-made rules, not heart-changing rules. As you examine your church assemblies, you can't tell sometimes what people have built upon. It looks like a house; all the houses look alike at first. But when this storm of judgment comes, there will be houses that will collapse. They have no solid foundation and are built on the sand. We must warn everyone—judgment is coming! It scares me to think that I could have missed or ignored the message of the credit card and the broken nails.

After I got off my knees, I had the words to a love song that says there's a holiness and a spirit-dove, a jealousy and a secret love. When God blows you a kiss in the form of long-awaited blessings or cross-felt suffering and disciplining, remember—judgment is now, and heaven is calling for the love that is due. I pray that no one misses it.

HEAVEN'S KISS[1]

There's a holiness and a bath of love / There's a beating heart from up above / There's a jealousy that I can't deny / There's a spirit-dove that you cannot buy

There's a time and place for every man / And our God will walk with us in this land / He's not far away for this is His plan / And He holds our hearts sweetly in His hands

There's a hungriness in my longing heart / A filling mystery found in the cross / And when heaven calls for the love that's due / I just blow that kiss right back to You

CHORUS: Holiness and spirit-dove / Jealousy and secret love / Be still my friend so you don't miss / What I call heaven's kiss

What You Can Do Today

- *Go where God is leading you in Scripture.*

- *Make a list of some ways that you can keep the flame of love for God alive in your heart.* Jesus warned that in the end times, the love of most would grow cold. How can you demonstrate to Him your love and devotion?

- *Begin to be very aware of when things seem to be going wrong for you.* Do you have any personal connections with God that can reveal the state of your relationship with Him (such as healthy fingernails, thriving boxwoods, etc.)? Is God trying to get your attention? Strive to be very attentive to His cues, and seek His Word when you feel you have fallen from His personal care.

- *Visualize how it would feel to have God turn His face completely away from you.* This complete emptiness would be the ultimate rejection. Starting now, do whatever is needed to grow closer to the Father and rejoice in His closeness!

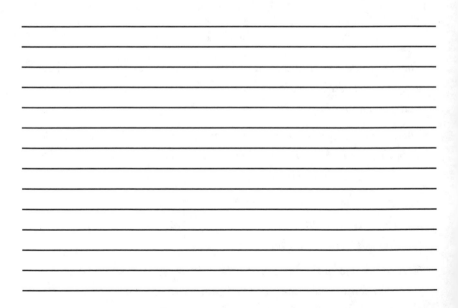

I'm Not Hungry Anymore

"Then Jesus declared, 'I am the bread of life. He who comes to me will never go hungry, and he who believes in me will never be thirsty'" (John 6:35). God is my morning and my night; He is my Alpha and Omega. He is the Beginning and the End. God is my everything and He is your everything, but you might not know that yet. There is nothing that He can't do, and He wants to show you if you would only give Him the floor for a few minutes. I learn something new every week. I am going to start a list of the things that He has been to me and for me, and you can add to it. I am not thirsty or hungry anymore because . . .

> *God is a mechanic. He can fix my car, computer, or camera.*
> *God is a roofer. He can fix my leaky roof without the help of*
> *human hands.*
> *God is my husband-defender. If my husband is not present,*
> *God can help me to the car with a heavy load and protect*
> *me. God is a conversationalist when I am alone, and He*
> *meets every need, in more ways than a spouse could do.*
> *God is my interior decorator. He can pick out colors, furniture,*
> *and paintings. My whole house is a result of calling upon*
> *Him for everything.*
> *God is my best friend. I used to try to give someone else this*
> *position, but I've learned through experience that there is*
> *no friend like Jesus.*
> *God is my business CEO. The more I consult Him, the better*
> *things go.*
> *God is my avenger. I never have to take revenge or get back*
> *at anyone.*
> *God is my clothing consultant. He puts my outfits together in*
> *the morning. When I pray, He makes great new things*
> *come to mind.*

God is my party coordinator. When I pray that people will have a good time, enjoy the food and company, and leave uplifted, the party is always great.

God is my only alarm clock. I have not set a mechanical one in years, and God has always awakened me one way or another. I start talking to Him first thing every day and thank Him for waking me. The rest of the day follows suit.

God is my primary songwriter and musician.

God is the journalist and Bible scholar of all my writings. I just let the Word fall open, and the rest is history.

God is my foremost entertainer. He always shows me something new.

God is the great chef. I pray over food; I want each flavor to be savored. Since God made everyone's taste buds, He knows how to provide everyone's favorite tastes.

God is my primary physician. I consult Him first for all things. Occasionally, He will refer me to other doctors.

God is my sure Savior from temptation because He has offered Himself to be the object of my affection.

God is my invisible traffic director. He can part great seas of heavy traffic.

When God is your everything, you think twice about loving any other sensation on this earth!

God is . . .

Appendix A

PHYSIOLOGICAL

There are several important steps involved in the process of transferring your heart from food to God. One is to confine your eating to the boundaries of hunger and fullness. To do this, you must learn to recognize the difference between true physiological hunger and head 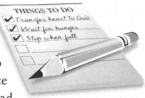 hunger. Physiological hunger is the *signal* God gave us to tell us when to eat, and this hunger can be satisfied only with *food*. Head hunger is the *desire* to eat regardless of true physiological hunger. It can also indicate an emptiness that we feel that can be satisfied only by *God*. As you begin to feed your body only when it is physiologically hungry, the amount you eat will be reduced dramatically, and you will lose weight. As this process continues, you will discover that eating when you are physiologically hungry is far more satisfying than eating for any other reason. God created food to be used as fuel, not as a comforter. The hunger signal is the only legitimate reason to eat. Your heart will begin to desire less and less food, and the old magnetism to it will begin to diminish.

STOMACH HUNGER

In The Weigh Down Workshop[†], we refer to physiological hunger as stomach hunger. It is an empty, hollow, burning sensation, which may be followed by a growl. The stomach is located above the waistline just under the rib cage, so don't confuse stomach growls with abdominal noises, which may be the result of overeating! Stomach hunger comes at different intervals after your last meal, depending upon what and how much was eaten and upon your activity level. Do not be impatient. Trust that your body knows when and how much it needs, and rely on it to signal you when it needs to be refueled. If you begin to doubt that your body has these signals, remember that they were perfectly intact at birth. When you were hungry, you ate, and when you were full, you stopped, and when you were sleepy, you slept. As you grew older, your natural hunger mechanism became unplugged as you followed man-made rules for eating, obeyed family table rules for cleaning your plate, and relied on diets and food exchanges to tell you what and when to eat. It is still intact, but you will need to be very sensitive to its cues at first. Keep waiting longer and eating smaller amounts until you discover the stomach growl.

Stopping when you are satisfied is as important as waiting for the hunger signal to eat. This is crucial to losing your excess weight, and it will be the single most active step you take toward letting go of greed—the key to permanent weight loss. While you are losing weight, do not be surprised if your body signals satisfaction after only a few bites. This is not at all unusual because your body is actually trying to use up its stored fat. It does not want another large meal to burn up before it is allowed to use the reserve fuel. In fact, the body uses food just as a car uses gas. Our hunger and fullness gauge is like the gas gauge on a car. "Empty" signals the need to refuel. "Full" signals enough. As long as your body has stored fuel, all it wants is a spark to keep the engine running so that it can burn what is stored. If you do overeat, do not despair—your body will once again signal you when it needs to be refueled. If overeating is habitual, then you are still grabbing more than your allotted share and not learning to be satisfied with the appropriate amount for your body. An occasional slip is no reason to give up and binge. Just start over, waiting for your hunger signal before you eat again.

Eating between the boundaries of hunger and fullness will automatically limit your food intake, sometimes as much as 75 percent. You will probably be amazed at how much more you had been eating than your body actually needed. It will come as no surprise, then, that you begin to lose weight as a result of eating smaller amounts. You

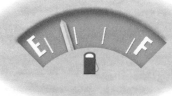

will also discover that these reduced amounts automatically result in lower fat, calorie, carbohydrate, and cholesterol intake. You do not have to keep track of these things at all! The more you continue eating reduced amounts, the greater satisfaction you will receive from what you are eating. Eventually, your desire for food outside the boundaries of hunger and fullness will go away.

One more thing to know as you begin this new way of eating is how important it is to *wait* for true stomach hunger before you eat. You see, God created such an efficient system that your body knows when it has too much fuel in reserve. The last meal you ate will be the first fuel that is used up. Then, the body will use up some of the stored fat *before* it signals hunger again. It is actually *designed* to rid itself of the stored fuel! Therefore, it is very important that you wait for that unquestionable hunger signal before you consume any more food. If you don't, you are not allowing your body to use the reserves (stored fat). You might maintain your present weight by doing this, but you won't lose any. For more in-depth information, call The Weigh Down Workshop† at 1-800-844-5208 to attend a seminar/support group near you.

HEAD HUNGER

In The Weigh Down Workshop†, all hunger other than true physiological hunger is defined as *head hunger*. In other words, head hunger is the desire for food *beyond* what the body is calling for. It includes going to food when we are stressed, angry, bored, sad, lonely, or lazy. But it also includes going to food just because it smells good, or because it looks good, or simply because it is there! Head hunger includes continuing to eat past full just because the food tastes good and is still on your plate. Head hunger also includes eating according to the clock, whether you are hungry or not. It is very important as you return to the process of eating according to hunger and fullness that you bypass eating with your family if you aren't truly hungry. Instead, sit with them as they eat, and enjoy mealtime as a time of togetherness. Visit with your family as you wait for your body to signal hunger. And the microwave oven makes it easy to eat later if your hunger didn't coincide with mealtime.

As you grow more familiar with this plan for eating, you will be able to adjust your hunger schedule very easily in just a few days, so that hunger will occur at mealtimes.

EXERCISE

Just as dieting does not help your heart desire less food, neither does exercising. Exercise does have virtue for physical fitness. There is no substitute for exercise when it comes to muscle toning, cardiovascular conditioning, and bone strengthening. It can also help with digestion and with the healthy function of your organs: "For physical training is of some value, but godliness has value for all things, holding promise for both the present life and the life to come" (1 Tim. 4:8). Exercise is great for physical training, but it does not help your heart desire less food or lessen the desire to control the food. Your goal is to get your focus off food, but it is very tempting to feel the need to stay "in control" by walking around the block or running several miles after a meal. If exercise has become a stronghold for you and causes a deeper self-focus, if you wake up every morning planning your entire day around your exercise routine, or if exercise is the only thing that gives you peace, then it is a false god in your life. Your goal should be to focus all of your heart, soul, mind, and strength onto God instead of food and your body. Trust God, not exercise—He is jealous of our misplaced dependence. The only exercise you require is getting down on your knees to pray and getting the muscle of your will to surrender control of your natural, God-given hunger and fullness guide to the Creator. The muscles of your eyes need to be fixed on Jesus Christ, and the muscle of your self-will needs to bow before the Father.

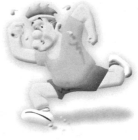

HELPFUL HINTS

- Eat only when you feel physiological hunger.
- Eat regular foods.
- If necessary, start by cutting your food amounts in half.
- Rate the food on your plate and eat the most pleasing bites first.

- Savor the taste of each bite.

- Stop as soon as you are satisfied.

- Rejoice in how little it takes to satisfy (instead of how much you can get away with).

- Eat more slowly.

- Eat with a fork; put it down between bites.

- When eating with others, enjoy the companionship as well as the food.

- If you have leftovers, save them for later or just throw them away. *Do not eat beyond full.*

- In a restaurant, ask for a carryout and take the rest of your great meal home. *Again, do not eat beyond full.*

- If you are tempted to continue eating after you are full, remove your plate from the table, cover it with a napkin, or leave the table.

- Drink water, tea, coffee, or noncaloric (diet) beverages between hunger periods.

- Avoid drinking sweetened beverages between hungers. The sugar will interfere with your sensing true hunger.

- Just as you eat when you are hungry, drink when you are thirsty.

- Notice that when you are really hungry, food tastes great! But the taste will diminish as hunger begins to be satisfied.

- If you overeat, simply wait for the next hunger signals before eating again.

- When you are tempted or challenged, go to God for your strength and your direction, and look only to Him as the object of your redirected passion. You will need something to love and adore, and only God can return this love.

EATING SITUATIONS

Many times, questions arise concerning the way to handle specific eating situations when you are trying to lose weight. The wonderful truth about losing weight the Weigh Down† way is that there are no special food rules to follow that include weighing, measuring, counting, or restricting food selections. *All* foods are to be enjoyed with thanksgiving between the boundaries

of hunger and fullness. The only rule is to get your heart right with God—
the body will follow. Listed here are some typical eating occasions and how
to handle them within the boundaries of hunger and fullness:

- *It is lunch hour and you are not hungry.* Don't eat. Your body is not calling for food, and if you do eat, it will only be added to what needs to
  be burned (your stored fat). If you get hungry before the next meal,
  you can eat a small snack of some kind to satisfy your hunger until
  mealtime—or you can choose to make *that* your mealtime.

- *You are about to starve, and mealtime is still an* hour *away.* Don't panic.
  Just drink an ounce or two of juice or eat something very small. This
  will satisfy your hunger enough to allow you to make it to mealtime.
  And even if you aren't able to eat a snack, just remember that this
  hunger *won't* kill you. In fact, the gnawing sensation will usually go
  away after a few minutes and won't come around again for a while,
  maybe an hour. Just don't use the premature hunger as an excuse to
  eat two meals!

- *You have only ten minutes to eat.* Then eat in ten minutes. The Weigh
  Down Workshop† recommends that you learn to slow down your
  eating for two reasons. First, you will be able to taste each bite
  instead of inhaling it. You can savor the quality instead of quantity.
  Second, you remain in much better control and can detect fullness
  better when you eat more slowly. The body processes food more
  slowly than the mouth chews it and swallows it. Therefore, it is
  important to eat slowly enough that your brain can signal your
  mouth that your stomach is full! However, once you have adjusted to
  the smaller amounts that your body is calling for, it is much easier to
  stop at a certain quantity, even if it has to be consumed in a short
  period of time. You must use all of these suggestions with the good
  judgment that God gave you and your body.

- *You hate breakfast and love midnight snacks.* No problem—as long as
  you are responding to hunger and fullness. You could be a "P.M. Person"
  who loves to sleep late and stay up late. These people usually start
  their day without hunger and prefer most of their food later in the day.
  Eating late at night is not wrong as long as you are hungry. And it
  stands to reason that if you eat late, you will probably not wake up
  hungry. The reverse is the "A.M. Person" who rises early, ready to eat.

These people often prefer heavier food early in the day, dwindling to lighter and less food at night. Either one is okay as long as you are using your hunger/fullness mechanism as your signal to eat.

You are satisfied, but there is still food on your plate. If you are at home, you can cover it and save it for later, or you can throw it away! If you are eating in a restaurant, you can leave it on your plate, or you can ask for a carryout and take it home. We have the misconception that it is wrong to leave food on the plate, but that is a myth perpetuated by some parents. The problem is *greed*—whether it is helping yourself to too much or eating too much. If you serve yourself and later realize that "your eyes were bigger than your stomach," learn to serve yourself smaller portions. If someone else prepares your plate, whether it is at home or in a restaurant, he has no idea how much you are hungry for and may bring you too much. You don't have to eat food just because it is there. Eat until you are satisfied, and either save or dispose of the rest. It's simple.

THE THIN EATER

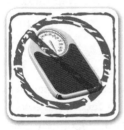

This is the thin person you have always known and envied because it seemed that he could eat so much wonderful food and never gain an ounce! You have always wanted to know his secret, or you thought that God just gave him a higher metabolism than yours. The truth is that he *does* eat whatever he "wants"—but he "wants" to eat *only when he is hungry*. What he "wants" is a small amount of food. Watch him over a forty-eight-hour period. He may skip some meals and may eat some large meals, but he does not overeat within that forty-eight-hour period. He does not binge eat. He eats larger volumes at some meals and smaller volumes at other meals because his intake is dictated *entirely* by hunger. If he eats more at times, he doesn't feel guilty because it was truly what his body was calling for. He doesn't even think about food again until he is hungry. He *enjoys* waiting until he is hungry to eat because the food tastes better. And the truth is that he may eat more than you do when you finally stop bingeing and join Weigh Down† because his body has no reserves (stored fat) that need to be burned up first. He burns his fuel from meal to meal. Once you have allowed your body to burn its reserves, your intake will also increase, or you may sense true hunger more often during the day because you no longer have stored fat cells or energy to burn. Just remember that eating when you are not hungry (when your body is not calling for it) is what causes excess weight—for *anyone*.

IDEAL BODY WEIGHT

God designed all of us along the same principles, but each body is quite unique. What is the ideal body weight for one person is not the ideal body weight for another. He designed our systems so efficiently that when you eat according to hunger and fullness, your body will naturally go to a slender size and remain there. Your body knows when its reserves have all been used up, and your hunger sensation either will come more often or will require more food before being satisfied. It is important not to focus on a specific weight. It is also important not to repeatedly skip hunger signs. Ignoring the signal that your body needs to eat is as disobedient as overeating. It can lead to anorexia and trying to maintain a body weight that is too thin and not healthy. As long as you are obedient to hunger and fullness, your body *will* reach and maintain the weight that God intends for you.

"VIRTUOUS" VITAMINS AND VEGETABLES

What about all those food rules concerning protein, vitamins, fats, calories, carbohydrates, basic four food groups, free foods, trigger foods, and so on? We have spent millions of dollars and years of research trying to figure out how the body functions and why it gains weight. But God never intended for us to worry about what we should eat and what we should drink—any more than He intended for us to worry about how much oxygen the body is getting in order to breathe (Matt. 6:25–27; Mark 7:14–19). He created a system that works automatically, without our even thinking about it. When we eat according to hunger and fullness, one of the things we discover is that the body has the amazing and very accurate ability to sense what it needs. It will alert us to that need *well* before it breaks down or becomes ill. All food groups do not need to be consumed in one day. The body *stores* nutrients, including vitamins, from the food just as a squirrel stores nuts for the winter. We also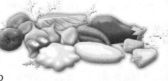

don't need to count calories or fat grams because the reduced amount of food that we are consuming (between hunger and fullness) will naturally reduce all those counts—calories, fat grams, carbohydrate grams, and so on.

The other misconception man has created is the idea that some foods are righteous and some foods are evil and can trigger an uncontrolled binge. *All foods are created to be received with thanksgiving* (1 Tim. 4:1–3). There will be consequences for *gluttony,* regardless of the appearance of righteousness or evil. *No* food is created to be eaten with greed, and the idea that a food is evil or forbidden often makes it overly tempting. When we continue to deny ourselves the wonderful food that God created for us because it contains fat grams, we are also sabotaging the system that He set up. He made fats to house flavor and aroma and created us to love both—but a little goes a long way. When we begin to add these satisfying foods back into our diet, remembering that hunger and fullness are our only boundaries, we discover that uncontrolled binges become things of the past.

HEALTH CONSIDERATIONS

It is always wise to consult your physician when making significant changes in your diet. If you are overweight, all physical ailments are greatly improved as a result of reducing your food intake, and the loss of excess weight improves your overall health. There are no special foods or medications required in this weight loss method. (Note: if you are currently taking medication that requires food, usually two or three ounces of juice or milk or a couple of crackers are sufficient. The stomach merely needs a buffer for protection against irritation caused by medications. Consult your physician.)

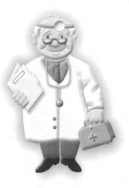

People with conditions such as diabetes, hypoglycemia, heart disease, certain food allergies, or other conditions usually associated with food restrictions have all been able to lose weight successfully following the principles taught in The Weigh Down Workshop†. Even the diabetic who has to eat at certain intervals can reduce the amount of food intake (and eventually insulin). This book helps to end the head hunger in the evening hours.

Pregnant and nursing mothers can lose weight following these guidelines because of the genius system God created. The pregnant and nursing woman's body knows its needs and will signal her accordingly. Eating what the body is calling for according to hunger and fullness ensures that both mother *and* baby will get everything they need. Many healthy babies have been delivered by Weigh Down† mothers. (For more information on pregnancy, lactation, and feeding infants and children, call 1-800-844-5208 to order *Feeding Children Physically and Spiritually.*)

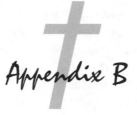

Appendix B

SPIRITUAL

The journey away from the pull of food is much like the Old Testament story about the journey the Israelites took out of Egypt, into the desert where their faithfulness was tested, and finally into the Promised Land of milk and honey.

EXODUS JOURNEY

The book of Exodus tells of how God's children, once subjugated to Pharaoh, were forced into slave labor to build temples and pyramids—towering icons to his sovereignty and power. Where they were once free men in a foreign land, they had become slaves, making bricks for Egypt. God heard their cries and began a mighty battle for their deliverance. The way was not always easy. When things got tough, the children of God were often tempted to return to the beckoning familiarity of Egyptian slavery, and they often questioned God's ability to take care of them (Ex. 14:10–12; 16:2–3; 17:1–3; Num. 11:4–6; 14:2–4). Because of this, they wandered for forty years in a desert that should never have taken that long to cross. In fact, most of them died in the desert, and it was their children who learned to trust God's love and wisdom and who finally entered the Promised Land (Num. 14:27–35). They experienced the peace and the happiness that can come only through submission to God—the One who loves us enough to discipline us and to demand obedience to His rules.

Our enslavement to food is similar. Where the Israelites were enslaved by Pharaoh and building monuments to his glory, we have worshiped food and elevated it to a place of unprecedented power in our lives. Our time has revolved so much around the contemplation, preparation, and consumption of food that it has become a continuous focus. Our hearts have been devoted to figuring out what the latest fad diet will or will not let us eat. The more we have focused on the food, the more control it has gained over us. Just as the Israelites crumbled under the weight of the bricks (Ex. 2:23b), we are crumbling under the weight of the food.

DESERT OF TESTING

When Moses—God's chosen leader—took the Israelites out of Egypt, he led them into the desert, where their faith in God was truly put to the test. They were challenged on all sides and were instructed to do many things that seemed contrary to reason (Ex. 15:22–25; 21:8–9). They had nothing other than their faith in God's sovereignty and His love for them as reassurance that their direction was true and that peace and freedom were at journey's end. However, the Israelites were slow to learn, and more than once, they questioned their leader, Moses; more than once, Moses questioned *his* leader, God Almighty (Num. 11:10–15, 21–22). They were forced to look to God for their basic needs, but God *always* delivered—and in miraculous ways! (Ex. 16:11–15; 17:1, 5–6).

In the same way, we must now follow God into the desert of testing, a place where we are told to get hungry before we eat, and to depend upon God to satisfy that hunger with just enough—not too much—food. We must now depend on the inside force of our God-given conscience. We no longer depend on the outside forces of our man-made diet rules. Despite their restrictions, those old rules are familiar to us and give us real boundaries; they are sometimes difficult to let go of. But each time we successfully follow God and are obedient to His direction, we are rewarded with a jewel such as weight loss, a smaller clothing size, or peace of mind and heart, and we are one step closer to the beauty and the freedom of the Promised Land.

PROMISED LAND

At the end of the desert journey, God's children entered the Promised Land (Josh. 3). This was the land that God had promised to the Israelites as the reward for their faithfulness (Ex. 3:17). Once they were there, their temptations diminished because they had learned to trust in God to provide for them. Their blessings were abundant. Again, the parallel is that once we are obedient to God in the area of eating, we not only lose the excess weight, but we lose the desire to overeat. What was once a temptation no longer plagues us, and we are free to live life without shame or a heavy heart. The excess weight does not return because we no longer have the *desire* to overeat.

SPIRITUAL BATTLE

In the process of transferring your focus from food and dieting to God, there will be a mighty battle for your heart. This is where Satan comes in. He is jealous of our devotion to God, and his sole purpose is to steal our hearts from God and perpetuate our misery and discontentment (Luke 8:5, 11–12; 1 Peter 5:8). As long as Satan can distract us from our true direction, he can successfully keep us from victory in our desert journey. He will distract us with lies, excuses, temptations, temporary failures, stressful situations, and other challenges that complicate and confuse the path to freedom (John 8:42–44). It is important to recognize these distractions for what they are and to know that the battle is already won (1 John 3:8b; James 4:7). You must trust that God's ways are always right. If you focus on Him and do not allow Satan to distract you, you will see His mighty right hand come to rescue you.

FALSE GODS/STRONGHOLDS/EGYPT/PRISON

A false god is what you have devoted your attention and your heart to, and now it has begun to control you (James 1:14–15). The references in this book to strongholds, Egypt, and the prison all have the same connotation— they refer to being in the grip of a false god. The misconception is that devotion to this false god will be fulfilling. But the truth is that devotion to *anything* other than God will ultimately be shallow and unfulfilling. It may provide temporary satisfaction, but eventually, a false god will take over your mind, your day, and your heart. Anything can become a false god— food, alcohol, cigarettes, television, pride, praise of men, love of money, love of power, sex, greed, work, anger, jealousy, or worry. The list goes on and on. Too often we want to attack the *object* of our devotion rather than our devotion to it. The truth is that food is not evil; sex is not evil; television is not evil; money is not evil. But our overwhelming *devotion* to and overindulgence in these things drive a wedge between us and the true fulfillment that can be given only by God. We can enjoy everything that God has given us, but we must adhere to His boundaries instead of continually grabbing for more than our share. It is *only* through God—not a false idol—that we will be truly filled. Psalm 24:4–5 states,

> *He who has clean hands and a pure heart,*
> *who does not lift up his soul to an idol*
> *or swear by what is false.*
> *He will receive blessing from the LORD*
> *and vindication from God his Savior.*

TRUE REPENTANCE

To be successful in overcoming any stronghold, we must first be honest with ourselves and with God. We cannot fix a problem until we admit that there is one! And the single greatest cause of our own grief is our lack of submission to God's will. He gave us a will and the freedom to choose whether or not we would obey Him (Deut. 30:19; Josh. 24:15). Sometimes we get caught up in the world's rules or in our own selfish desires, and we totally disregard the direction that God is leading us in because we think that something else will be better. But we are *never* right! We may feel temporary elation at our false victory, but eventually, the

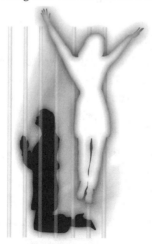

Father's wisdom is revealed (Eph. 1:17), and we feel only guilt and regret. God talks to us through that wonderful mechanism He created called the *conscience*. It is amazing how even the "smallest" or most "harmless" misdemeanors can spark a feeling of doubt or guilt in the mind or in the spirit—but we usually successfully ignore it and go on following our own wills. *True repentance* involves owning up to your idolatry, your greed, or your strong will, and laying it down for no other reason than the fact that it is outside God's will. True repentance desires nothing other than true obedience. It expects nothing in return. It is repentance for the sake of Christ because the activity or the behavior or the spirit is wrong (Acts 26:20). It is only when we reach true repentance that we can begin to experience the freedom and exhilaration of true deliverance. As God declares in Ezekiel 18:32b, "Repent and live!"

SUBMISSION

Submission is the act of yielding to the will of another. True submission involves no deals, no expectations, and no compromises. Even Jesus offered His prayers to God in reverent submission (Heb. 5:7). God desires that we be totally submissive to Him and to His will for us. The marital relationship is one example God uses to teach us submission. A wife is to be submissive to her husband, and the husband is to love his wife (Eph. 5:22–33). To submit means you do not always insist upon getting your way or going the direction you want to go. True submission to God and His will results in an inner peace regardless of the outward circumstances. Inevitably, you realize that God's wisdom *far* exceeds your own. In the end, you will see that His way is always better than your ways, and the blessings you receive from submitting to His will are always greater than anything you could grab for yourself.

WAYS OF ESCAPE

Many times we are faced with situations on the desert journey where we are really tempted to eat beyond our need. The wonderful thing is that there was a time when we didn't even recognize these as temptations. Now

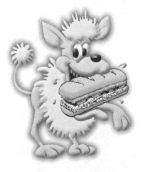

we can distinguish them for what they are— and we can handle them. God promises to provide us a way out or a "way of escape" from these temptations (1 Cor. 10:13). We used to call some ways of escape just "coincidences," such as going to the freezer for ice cream only to discover that it is covered with freezer burn or even completely gone! Some ways of escape are funny, such as struggling to open the microwave popcorn bag, only to have the bag

tear and scatter popcorn all over the kitchen floor! Or going to great lengths
to prepare a large double-decker submarine sandwich, only to find it in the
dog's mouth after stepping out to take a phone call. As you begin to recognize God's ways of escape, remember that He is looking for your willful *obedience,* not just your dependence upon Him to bail you out of temptations.
But when He knows your heart is devoted to Him, He is very faithful to
provide you with a way out.

JEWELS

The only sure path to freedom through the desert of testing is following
God's guidance the whole way. Sometimes the way is clear, and obedience
is not difficult. Other times we are tempted by Satan to follow his path
instead, which is filled with immediate gratification, temporary pleasure,
and false promises. But every time we bypass Satan's trap and steadfastly
cling to God and His truth, He rewards our effort with *jewels.* Jewels come
in many forms. A jewel may be something as simple as the feeling of accom-
plishment that comes from being obedient to God. It may be as complex as
seeing a whole chain of events come together and result in a positive conclusion. A jewel could be intangible, for example, an unexpected compliment from a friend or coworker, or it could be something tangible, such as
a smaller dress size. A jewel may be immediate, or it may be long in coming, but God's timing is always perfect! The key is to trust God completely.
He does not bring us into the desert to abandon us. He brings us to the
desert to test us and to strengthen our faith in Him so that we can see His
mighty right hand rescue us. As you turn away from the food and give your
wholehearted devotion to God Almighty, be attentive and watchful, and
you will recognize the wonderful jewels He is sending your way!

Notes

CHAPTER 1 — A PASSIONATE PEOPLE

1. "Position of the American Dietetic Association: Weight Management," *Journal of the American Dietetic Association,* vol. 97, January 1997, 71–74.

CHAPTER 2 — AMERICA HAS A CRUSH ON FOOD

1. "Most Americans Are Overweight," *Nutrition Guide,* American Heart Association, www.heartinfo.org.
2. "Position of the American Dietetic Association: Weight Managment," *Journal of the American Dietetic Association,* vol. 97, January 1997, 71–74.
3. "Obesity Gaining Ground," *Healthy Kids,* June/July 1999.
4. "Questions and Answers About Obesity," American Heart Association, June 1998.

CHAPTER 4 — THE WEIGH DOWN† EXPLOSION

1. *NBC Nightly News,* MSNBC, July 26, 1999.

CHAPTER 6 — SECRET OF THE PRISON

1. "Diagnosis: Miracle," *Tennessean,* September 23, 1998.

CHAPTER 8 — HUNGER IN THE DESERT

1. "Dealing with the Depths of Depression," U.S. Food and Drug Administration, *FDA Consumer Magazine,* July/August 1998.
2. Eleanor Noss Whitney and Sharon Rady Rolfes, *Understanding Nutrition,* 7th ed. (St. Paul: West Publishing Company, 1996).

CHAPTER 9 — SAVE YOUR HEART FOR ME

1. "Save Your Heart for Me," 1963 Polygram International Publishing, Inc. (ASCAP), Warner Bros. Music (ASCAP), Andrew Scott, Inc. (ASCAP). Written by Gary Geld and Peter Udell.

CHAPTER 12 — INNOCENT IN HIS SIGHT

1. "Drugs and Crime Facts," U.S. Department of Justice, Bureau of Justice Statistics, *Compendium of Federal Justice Statistics,* 1996.
2. Health and Human Services Annual Household Survey, *Tennessean,* August 19, 1999.
3. "Deaths Due to Alcohol," *Scientific American,* December 1996.
4. "Annual National Drug Survey Results Released," U.S. Department of Health and Human Services, August 17, 1999.
5. "Baseball and Tobacco: Spittin' Image," *Miami Herald,* July 1993.
6. "Position of the American Dietetic Association: Weight Managment," *Journal of the American Dietetic Association,* vol. 97, January 1997, 71–74.
7. "Virginia Officials Fight Growth of Adult Video Industry," *Washington Post,* July 25, 1997.
8. LDS.NET (Latter-Day Saint News), February 2, 1999.
9. *Body Doubles: The Twin Experience,* produced by Antony Thomas in association with Carlton Television and Home Box Office, 1997.

CHAPTER 13 — THE REMNANT

1. Henry H. Halley, *Halley's Bible Handbook: An Abbreviated Bible Commentary,* 24th ed. (Grand Rapids: Zondervan, 1965).
2. "Easter Draws Americans Back to Church," Gallup News Service, April 2, 1999.

CHAPTER 14 — HEAVEN'S KISS

1. "Heaven's Kiss," 1999 Weigh Down[†] Publishing (SESAC). Administered by Gwen Shamblin and The Weigh Down Workshop[†], Inc. Written by Gwen Shamblin.

Where Two or More Are Gathered...

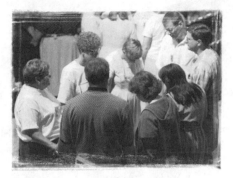

Enjoy the love and support of others traveling the road from slavery to the Promised Land.

- Join one of 30,000 groups meeting weekly in 50 states and 70 countries.

- Two 12-week seminars to choose from—**EXODUS Out of Egypt** (for weight loss) and **EXODUS from Strongholds** (helping participants break free from other destructive habits and deep-rooted problems).

- No embarrassing weigh-ins—just encouragement from others who are being set free from the desire to overeat.

- Receive your own 180-page workbook and 12 audiocassettes.

- Instructional videos featuring Gwen Shamblin.

- Encouraging testimonies from people who have lost 15 to 180 pounds.

- Experience permanent weight loss as you are set free from all destructive strongholds—discover a closer, more vibrant relationship with God.

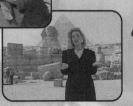

- Achieve a change of heart and behavior rather than attempting to lose weight by changing your environment and the content of food, taking pills, using liquid fasts, or exercising excessively.

For a class location near you, call, write, or visit our Web site!

Weigh Down Workshop[†]
P.O. Box 689099 • Franklin, TN 37068-9099
Phone (800) 844-5208 • Fax (800) 340-2142
www.wdworkshop.com

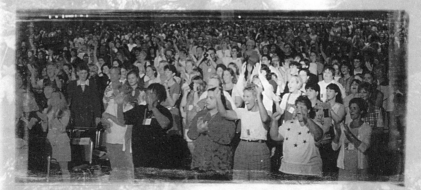

Experience Desert Oasis Each Summer in Nashville!

Gwen Shamblin invites you to join her and thousands of people from around the world for a powerful time of encouragement, teaching, praise, and amazing testimonies at Desert Oasis. It is a powerful, Spirit-filled event drawing you closer to our heavenly Father! For more information about each year's event, call us at **800-844-5208** or visit us on-line at **www.wdworkshop.com**.

Visit our Web site regularly for all the latest Weigh Down†
news and information. Find us at **www.wdworkshop.com**.